Use R!

Use R!

This series of inexpensive and focused books on R will publish shorter books aimed at practitioners. Books can discuss the use of R in a particular subject area (e.g., epidemiology, econometrics, psychometrics) or as it relates to statistical topics (e.g., missing data, longitudinal data). In most cases, books will combine LaTeX and R so that the code for figures and tables can be put on a website. Authors should assume a background as supplied by Dalgaard's Introductory Statistics with R or other introductory books so that each book does not repeat basic material.

More information about this series at http://www.springer.com/series/6991

Robin Genuer · Jean-Michel Poggi

Random Forests with R

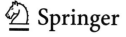 Springer

Robin Genuer
ISPED
University of Bordeaux
Bordeaux, France

Jean-Michel Poggi
Lab. Maths Orsay (LMO)
Paris-Saclay University
Orsay, France

ISSN 2197-5736   ISSN 2197-5744   (electronic)
Use R!
ISBN 978-3-030-56484-1   ISBN 978-3-030-56485-8   (eBook)
https://doi.org/10.1007/978-3-030-56485-8

This Springer imprint is published by the registered company Springer Nature Switzerland AG
The registered company address is: Gewerbestrasse 11, 6330 Cham, Switzerland

Preface

Random forests are a statistical learning method introduced by Leo Breiman in 2001. They are extensively used in many fields of application, due for sure not only to their excellent predictive performance, but also to their flexibility, with a few restrictions on the nature of the data. Indeed, random forests are adapted to both supervised classification problems and regression problems. In addition, they allow to consider qualitative and quantitative explanatory variables together without preprocessing. Moreover, they can be used to process standard data for which the number of observations is higher than the number of variables, while also performing very well in the high dimensional case, where the number of variables is quite large in comparison to the number of observations. Consequently, they are now among preferred methods in the toolbox of statisticians and other data scientists.

Who Is This Book for?

This book is an application-oriented statistical presentation of random forests. It is therefore primarily intended not only for students in academic fields such as statistical education, but also for practitioners in statistics and machine learning. A scientific undergraduate degree is quite sufficient to take full advantage of the concepts, methods, and tools covered by the book. In terms of computer science skills, little background knowledge is required, though an introduction to the R language is recommended.

Book Content

Random forests are part of the family of tree-based methods; accordingly, after an introductory chapter, Chap. 2 presents CART trees. The next three chapters are devoted to random forests. They focus on their presentation (Chap. 3), on the variable importance tool (Chap. 4), and on the variable selection problem (Chap. 5), respectively.

The structure of the chapters (except the introduction) is always the same. After a presentation of the concepts and methods, we illustrate their implementation on a running example. Then, various complements are provided before examining additional examples.

Throughout the book, each result is given together with the R code that can be used to reproduce it. All lines of code are available online[1] making things easy.

Thus, the book offers readers essential information and concepts, together with examples and the software tools needed to analyze data using random forests.

Orsay, France   Robin Genuer
June 2020   Jean-Michel Poggi

---

[1]https://RFwithR.robin.genuer.fr.

Acknowledgements

Our first thanks go to Eva Hiripi who suggested the idea of publishing the English version of the French original edition of the book entitled "Les forêts aléatoires avec R" (Presses Universitaires de Rennes Ed.).

We would like to thank our colleagues who shared our thoughts about these topics through numerous collaborations, in particular, Sylvain Arlot, Servane Gey, Christine Tuleau-Malot, and Nathalie Villa-Vialaneix.

We would also like to thank Nicolas Bousquet and Fabien Navarro who saved us a lot of time by providing us a first raw translation, thanks to the tool they developed for a large-scale automatic translation conducted in 2018. Of course, the authors are entirely responsible for the final translated version.

Finally, we thank three anonymous reviewers for their useful comments and insightful suggestions.

Contents

Chapter 1
Introduction to Random Forests with R

Abstract The two algorithms discussed in this book were proposed by Leo Breiman: CART trees, which were introduced in the mid-1980s, and random forests, which emerged just under 20 years later in the early 2000s. This chapter offers an introduction to the subject matter, beginning with a historical overview. Some notations, used to define the various statistical objectives addressed in the book, are also introduced: classification, regression, prediction, and variable selection. In turn, the three R packages used in the book are listed, and some competitors are mentioned. Lastly, the four datasets used to illustrate the methods' application are presented: the running example (spam), a genomic dataset, and two pollution datasets (ozone and dust).

1.1 Preamble

The two algorithms discussed in this book were proposed by Leo Breiman: CART (Classification And Regression Trees) trees, which were introduced in the mid-1980s (Breiman et al. 1984), and random forests (Breiman 2001), which emerged just under 20 years later in the early 2000s. At the confluence of statistics and statistical learning, this shortcut among Leo Breiman's multiple contributions, whose scientific biography is described in Olshen (2001) and Cutler (2010), provides a remarkable figure of these two disciplines.

Decision trees are the basic tool for numerous tree-based ensemble methods. Although known for decades and very attractive because of their simplicity and interpretability, their use suffered, until the 1980s, from serious justified objections. From this point of view, CART offers to decision trees the conceptual framework of automatic model selection, giving them theoretical guarantees and broad applicability while preserving their ease of interpretation.

But one of the major drawbacks, instability, remains. The idea of random forests is to exploit the natural variability of trees. More specifically, it is a matter of disrupting the construction by introducing some randomness in the selection of both individuals and variables. The resulting trees are then combined to construct the final prediction, rather than choosing one of them. Several algorithms based on such principles have thus been developed, for many of them, by Breiman himself: Bagging (Breiman 1996), several variants of the Arcing (Breiman 1998), and Adaboost (Freund and Schapire 1997).

Random forests (RF in the following) are therefore a nonparametric method of statistical learning widely used in many fields of application, such as the study of microarrays (Díaz-Uriarte and Alvarez De Andres 2006), ecology (Prasad et al. 2006), pollution prediction (Ghattas 1999), and genomics (Goldstein et al. 2010; Boulesteix et al. 2012), and for a broader review, see Verikas et al. (2011). This universality is first and foremost linked to excellent predictive performance. This can be seen in Fernández-Delgado et al. (2014) which crowns RF in a recent large-scale comparative evaluation, whereas less than a decade earlier, the article in Wu et al. (2008) with similar objectives mentions CART but not yet random forests! In addition, they are applicable to many types of data. Indeed, it is possible to consider high-dimensional data for which the number of variables far exceeds the number of observations. In addition, they are suitable for both classification problems (categorical response variable) and regression problems (continuous response variable). They also allow handling a mixture of qualitative and quantitative explanatory variables. Finally, they are, of course, able to process standard data for which the number of observations is greater than the number of variables.

Beyond the performance and the easy to tune feature of the method with very few parameters to adjust, one of the most important aspects in terms of application is the quantification of the explanatory variables' relative importance. This concept, which is not so much examined by statisticians (see, for example, Grömping 2015, in regression), finds a convenient definition in the context of random forests that is easy to evaluate and which naturally extends to the case of groups of variables (Gregorutti et al. 2015).

Therefore, and we will emphasize this aspect very strongly, RF can be used for variable selection. Thus, in addition to a powerful prediction tool, it can also be used to select the most interesting explanatory variables to explain the response, among a potentially very large number of variables. This is very attractive in practice because it helps both to interpret more easily the results and, above all, to determine influential factors for the problem of interest. Finally, it can also be beneficial for prediction, because eliminating many irrelevant variables makes the learning task easier.

1.2 Notation

Throughout the book, we will adopt the following notations. We assume that a learning sample is available:

$$\mathcal{L}_n = \{(X_1, Y_1), \ldots, (X_n, Y_n)\}$$

composed of n couples of independent and identically distributed observations, coming from the same common distribution as a couple (X, Y). This distribution is, of course, unknown in practice and the purpose is precisely to estimate it, or more specifically to estimate the link that exists between X and Y.

We call the coordinates of X the "input variables" (or "explanatory variables" or "variables"), where we note X^j for the jth coordinate, and we assume that $X \in \mathcal{X}$, a certain space that we will specify later. However, we assume that this space is of dimension p, where p is the (total) number of variables.

Y refers to the "response variable" (or "explained variable" or "dependent variable") and $Y \in \mathcal{Y}$. The nature of the regression or classification problem depends on the nature of the space $\mathcal{Y}$:

- If $\mathcal{Y} = \mathbb{R}$, we have a regression problem.
- If $\mathcal{Y} = \{1, \ldots, C\}$, we have a classification problem with C classes.

1.3 Statistical Objectives

Prediction

The first learning objective is prediction. We are trying, using the learning sample $\mathcal{L}_n$, to construct a predictor:

$$\widehat{h} : \mathcal{X} \to \mathcal{Y}$$

which associates a prediction $\widehat{y}$ of the response variable corresponding to any given input observation $x \in \mathcal{X}$.

The "hat" on $\widehat{h}$ is a notation to specify that this predictor is constructed using $\mathcal{L}_n$. We omit the dependence over n for the predictor to simplify the notations, but it does exist.

More precisely, we want to build a powerful predictor in terms of prediction error (also called generalization error):

- In regression, we will consider here the mathematical expectation of the quadratic error: $\mathrm{E}\left[(Y - \widehat{h}(X))^2\right]$.
- In classification, the probability of misclassification: $\mathrm{P}\left(Y \neq \widehat{h}(X)\right)$.

The prediction error depends on the unknown joint distribution of the random couple (X, Y), so it must be estimated. One classical way to proceed is, using a test sample $\mathcal{T}_m = \{(X'_1, Y'_1), \ldots, (X'_m, Y'_m)\}$, also drawn from the distribution of (X, Y), to calculate an empirical test error:

- In regression, it is the mean square error: $\frac{1}{m} \sum_{i=1}^{m} \left(Y'_i - \widehat{h}(X'_i)\right)^2$.
- In classification, the misclassification rate: $\frac{1}{m} \sum_{i=1}^{m} \mathbf{1}_{Y'_i \neq \widehat{h}(X'_i)}$.

In the case where a test sample is not available, the prediction error can still be estimated, for example, by cross-validation. In addition, we will introduce later on a specific estimate using random forests.

Remark 1.1 In this book, we focus on regression problems and/or supervised classification ones. However, RF have been generalized to various other statistical problems.

First, for survival data analysis, Ishwaran et al. (2008) introduced Random Survival Forests, transposing the main ideas of RF to the case for which the quantity to be predicted is the time to event. Let us also mention on this subject the work of Hothorn et al. (2006).

Random forests have also been generalized to the multivariate response variable case (see the review by Segal and Xiao 2011, which also provides references from the 1990s).

Selection and importance of variables

A second classical objective is variable selection. This involves determining a subset of the input variables that are actually useful and active in explaining the input–output relationship. The quality of a subset of selected variables is often assessed by the performance obtained with a predictor using only these variables instead of all the initial sets.

In addition, we can focus on constructing a hierarchy of input variables based on a quantification of the importance of the effects on the output variable. Such an index of importance therefore provides a ranking of variables, from the most important to the least important.

1.4 Packages

We will mainly focus on R three packages (R Core Team 2018):

- **rpart** (Therneau and Atkinson 2018) for tree methods, in Chap. 2.
- **randomForest** (Liaw and Wiener 2018) for random forests, in Chaps. 3 and 4.
- **VSURF** (Genuer et al. 2018) for variable selection using random forests, in Chap. 5.

Remark 1.2 Regarding the variants of random forests discussed in the previous section, the **randomForestSRC** package (Ishwaran and Kogalur 2017) provides a unified implementation of RF for regression, supervised classification, in a survival context as well as for the multivariate response case.

1.5 Datasets

1.5.1 Running Example: Spam Detection

We will illustrate the application of the different methods on the very classical spam data for educational purposes, as a running example.

This well-known and freely available dataset is due to an engineer from Hewlett-Packard company, named George, who analyzed a sample of his professional emails:

- The observations are the 4,601 emails, of which 2,788 (i.e., 60 %) are desirable emails and 1,813 (i.e., 40 %) are undesirable emails, i.e., spam.
- The response variable is therefore binary: spam or non-spam. We will rename the category non-spam to ok to make some graphs easier to read.
- There are $p = 57$ explanatory variables: 54 are proportions of occurrences of words or characters, such as $ (denoted charDollar), ! (denoted charExclamation), free, money, and hp, two are related to the lengths of the capital letter sequences (the average, capitalAve, the longest, capitalLong), and finally the last is the number of capital letters in the mail, capitalTotal. These variables are classical and are defined using standard text analysis procedures, allowing observations characterized by texts to be statistically processed through numerical variables.

The statistical objectives stated above are formulated for this example as follows: first, we want to build a good spam filter: a new email arrives, we have to predict if it is spam or not. Secondly, we are also interested in knowing which variables are the most important for the spam filter (here, words or characters).

To assess the performance of a spam filter, the dataset is randomly split into two parts: 2,300 emails are used for learning while the other 2,301 emails are used to test predictions.[1]

So we have a problem of **2-class classification** ($C = 2$) with a number of individuals ($n = 2,300$ for learning, model building) much larger than the number of variables ($p = 57$). In addition, we have a large test sample ($m = 2,301$) to evaluate an estimate of the prediction error.

Let us load the dataset into R, available in the **kernlab** package (Karatzoglou et al. 2004); let us rename the category nonspam to ok and fix the learning and test sets:

---

[1] Other usual choices are 70% of data for learning, 30% for test or even 80–20%: we choose 50–50% to stabilize estimation errors and reduce computational times.

```
> data("spam", package = "kernlab")
> set.seed(9146301)
> levels(spam$type) <- c("ok", "spam")
> yTable <- table(spam$type)
> indApp <- c(sample(1:yTable[2], yTable[2]/2),
    sample((yTable[2] + 1):nrow(spam), yTable[1]/2))
> spamApp <- spam[indApp, ]
> spamTest <- spam[-indApp, ]
```

Remark 1.3 The command `set.seed(9146301)` allows fixing the seed of the random numbers generator in R. Thus, if the previous instruction block is executed several times, there will be no variability in the learning and test samples.

1.5.2 Ozone Pollution

The `Ozone` data is used in many papers and is one of the classical benchmark datasets since the article of Breiman and Friedman 1985.

The objective here is to predict the maximum ozone concentration associated with a day in 1976 in the Los Angeles area, using 12 weather and calendar variables. The data consist of 366 observations and 13 variables, each observation is associated with a day. The 13 variables are as follows:

- V1 Months: $1 =$ January, ..., $12 =$ December.
- V2 Day of the month 1 to 31.
- V3 Day of the week: $1 =$ Monday, ..., $7 =$ Sunday.
- V4 Daily maximum of hourly average of ozone concentrations.
- V5 500 millibar (*m*) pressure height measured at Vandenberg AFB.
- V6 Wind speed (*mph*) at Los Angeles International Airport (LAX).
- V7 Humidity (*%*) at LAX.
- V8 Temperature (*degrees F*) measured at Sandburg, California.
- V9 Temperature (*degrees F*) measured at El Monte, California.
- V10 Inversion base height (*feet*) at LAX.
- V11 Pressure gradient (*mmHg*) from LAX to Daggett, California.
- V12 Inversion base temperature (*degrees F*) to LAX.
- V13 Visibility (*miles*) measured at LAX.

So it is a problem of **regression** where we have to predict V4 (the daily maximum ozone concentration) using the other 12 variables, nine meteorological variables (V5 to V13), and three calendar variables (V1 to V3).

In many cases, only continuous explanatory variables are considered. Here, the tree methods allow all of them to be taken into account, even if including V2 the day of the month is a priori irrelevant.

This dataset is available in the `mlbench` package (Leisch and Dimitriadou 2010) and can be loaded into R using the following command:

```
> data("Ozone", package = "mlbench")
```

1.5.3 Genomic Data for a Vaccine Study

The dataset `vac18` is from an HIV prophylactic vaccine trial (Thiébaut et al. 2012). Expressions of a subset of 1,000 genes were measured for 42 observations corresponding to 12 negative HIV participants, from 4 different stimuli:

- The candidate vaccine (LIPO5).
- A vaccine containing the Gag peptide (GAG).
- A vaccine not containing the Gag peptide (GAG-).
- A non-stimulation (NS).

The prediction objective here is to determine, in view of gene expression, the stimulation that has been used. So it is a **4-class high-dimensional classification** problem. It should be noted that this prediction problem is an intermediate step in order to reach the actual objective which is the selection of the most useful genes for the discrimination between the different vaccines.

We load the `vac18` data, available in the `mixOmics` package (Le Cao et al. 2017):

```
> data("vac18", package = "mixOmics")
```

1.5.4 Dust Pollution

These data are published in Jollois et al. (2009).

Airborne particles come from various origins, natural or human-induced, and the chemical composition of these particles can vary a lot. In 2009, Air Normand, the air quality agency in Upper Normandy (Haute-Normandie), had about ten devices measuring the concentrations of PM10 particles of diameter of less than 10 μ/m, expressed in $\mu/g/m^3$, in average over the past quarter of an hour. European regulation rules set the value of 50 $\mu/g/m^3$ (as a daily average) as the limit not to exceed more than 35 days in the year for PM10.

We focused on a subnetwork of six PM10 monitoring stations: three in Rouen GCM (industrial), JUS (urban), and GUI (near traffic); two in Le Havre REP (traffic) and HRI (urban); and finally a rural station in Dieppe AIL.

The data considered for the six stations are

- For weather: rain PL, wind speed VV (max and average), wind direction DV (max and dominant), temperature T (min, max, and average), temperature gradient GT (Le Havre and Rouen), atmospheric pressure PA, and relative humidity HR (min, max, and average).
- For pollutants: dust (PM10), nitrogen oxides (NO, NO2) for urban pollution and sulfur dioxide (SO2) for industrial pollution: in addition to those measured at each station, pollutants measured nearby are added:
  - For GUI: addition of SO2 measured at JUS.
  - For REP: addition of SO2 measured in Le Havre (MAS station).
  - For HRI: addition of NO and NO2 measured at Le Havre (MAS station).

Let us load the data for the JUS station, included in the **VSURF** package:

```
> data("jus", package = "VSURF")
```

Chapter 2
CART

Abstract CART stands for Classification And Regression Trees, and refers to a statistical method for constructing tree predictors (also called decision trees) for both
regression and classification problems. This chapter focuses on CART trees, analyzing in detail the two steps involved in their construction: the maximal tree growing
algorithm, which produces a large family of models, and the pruning algorithm, which
is used to select an optimal or suitable final one. The construction is illustrated on
the spam dataset using the rpart package. The chapter then addresses interpretability issues and how to use competing and surrogate splits. In the final section, trees
are applied to two examples: predicting ozone concentration and analyzing genomic
data.

2.1   The Principle

CART stands for Classification And Regression Trees, and refers to a statistical
method, introduced by Breiman et al. (1984), for constructing tree predictors (also
called decision trees) for both regression and classification problems.

Let us start by considering a very simple classification tree on our running example
about spam detection (Fig. 2.1).

A CART tree is an upside-down tree: the root is at the top. The leaves of the tree
are the nodes without descendants (for this example, 5 leaves) and the other nodes
of the tree are nonterminal nodes (4 such nodes including the root) that have two
child nodes. Hence, the tree is said to be binary. Nonterminal nodes are labeled by a
condition (a question) and leaves by a class label or a value of the response variable.
When a tree is given, it is easy to use it for prediction. Indeed, to determine the
predicted value $\widehat{y}$ for a given x, it suffices to go through the only path from the root
to a leaf, by answering the sequence of questions given by the successive splits and
reading the value of y labeling the reached leaf. When you go through the tree, the
rule is as follows: if the condition is verified then you go to the left node and if not, go
to the right. In our example, an email with proportions of occurrences of characters
"!" and "$", respectively, larger than 7.95 and 0.65% will thus be predicted as spam
by this simple tree.

© Springer Nature Switzerland AG 2020   9
R. Genuer and J.-M. Poggi, *Random Forests with R*, Use R!,
https://doi.org/10.1007/978-3-030-56485-8_2

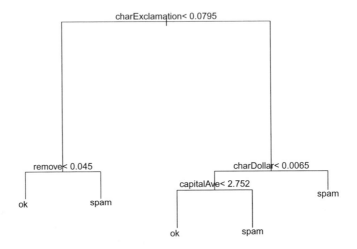

Fig. 2.1 A very simple first tree, spam data

Other methods for building decision trees, sometimes introduced before CART, are available, such as CHAID (Kass 1980) and C4.5 (Quinlan 1993). Tree methods are still of interest today, as can be seen in Patil and Bichkar (2012) in computer science and Loh (2014) in statistics. Several variants for building CART trees are possible, for example, by changing the family of admissible splits, the cost function, or the stopping rule. We limit ourselves in the sequel to the most commonly used variant, which is presented in Breiman et al. (1984). The latter contains many variants which have not been widely disseminated and implemented. Indeed, the success of the simplest version has been ensured by its ease of interpretation. A concise and clear presentation in French of the regression CART method can be found in Chap. 2 of Gey (2002) PhD thesis.

CART proceeds by recursive binary partitioning of the input space $\mathcal{X}$ and then determines an optimal sub-partition for prediction. Building a CART tree is therefore a two-step process. First, the construction of a maximal tree and the second step, called pruning, which builds a sequence of optimal subtrees pruned from the maximal tree sufficient from an optimization perspective.

2.2 Maximal Tree Construction

At each step of the partitioning process, a part of the space previously obtained is split into two pieces. We can therefore naturally associate a binary tree to the partition built step by step. The nodes of the tree correspond to the elements of the partition. For example, the root of the tree is associated with the entire input space, its two child nodes with the two subspaces obtained by the first split, and so on. Figure 2.2

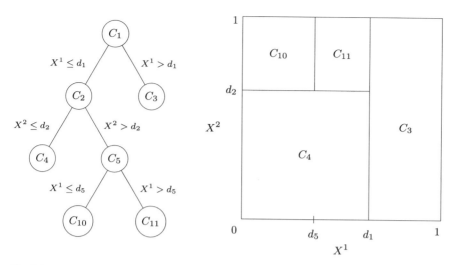

Fig. 2.2 Left: a classification tree to predict the class label corresponding to a given x. Right: the associated partition in the explanatory variables' space, here the unit square (C_1, C_2, and C_5 do not appear because they are not associated with leaves)

illustrates the correspondence between a binary tree and the associated partition of the explanatory variables' space (here the unit square).

Let us now detail the splitting rule. To make things simple, we limit to continuous explanatory variables while mentioning the qualitative case, whenever necessary. The input space is then $\mathbb{R}^p$, where p is the number of variables. Let us consider the root of the tree, associated with the entire space $\mathbb{R}^p$, which contains all the observations of the learning sample $\mathcal{L}_n$. The first step of CART is to optimally split this root into two child nodes, and then this splitting is repeated recursively in a similar way. We call a split an element of the form

$$\{X^j \leq d\} \cup \{X^j > d\},$$

where $j \in \{1, \ldots, p\}$ and $d \in \mathbb{R}$. Splitting according to $\{X^j \leq d\} \cup \{X^j > d\}$ means that all observations whose value of the jth variable is smaller than d go into the left child node, and all those whose value is larger than d go into the right child node. The method then looks for the best split, i.e., the couple (j, d) that minimizes a certain cost function:

- In the regression case, one tries to minimize the within-group variance resulting from splitting a node t into two child nodes t_L and t_R, the variance of a node t being defined by $V(t) = \frac{1}{\#t} \sum_{i:x_i \in t} (y_i - \bar{y}_t)^2$ where $\bar{y}_t$ and $\#t$ are, respectively, the average and the number of the observations y_i belonging to the node t. We are therefore seeking to maximize:

$$V(t) - \left(\frac{\#t_L}{\#t} V(t_L) + \frac{\#t_R}{\#t} V(t_R)\right).$$

- In the classification case, the possible labels are $\{1, \ldots, C\}$, and the impurity of the child nodes is most often quantified through the Gini index. The Gini index of a node t is defined by $\Phi(t) = \sum_{c=1}^{C} \hat{p}_t^c (1 - \hat{p}_t^c)$, where $\hat{p}_t^c$ is the proportion of observations of class c in the node t. We are then led, for any node t and any admissible split, to maximize

$$\Phi(t) - \left(\frac{\#t_L}{\#t} \Phi(t_L) + \frac{\#t_R}{\#t} \Phi(t_R)\right).$$

It should be emphasized that at each node, the search for the best split is made among all the variables. Thus, a variable can be used in several splits (or only one time or never).

In regression, we are therefore looking for splits that tend to reduce the variance of the resulting nodes. In classification, we try to decrease the Gini purity function, and thus to increase the homogeneity of the obtained nodes, a node being perfectly homogeneous if it contains only observations of the same class label. It should be noted that the homogeneity of the nodes could be measured by another function, such as the misclassification rate, but this natural choice does not lead to a strictly concave purity function guaranteeing the uniqueness of the optimum at each split. This property, while not absolutely essential from a statistical point of view, is useful from a computational point of view by avoiding ties for the best split selection.

In the case of a nominal explanatory variable X^j, the above remains valid except that in this case, a split is simply an element of the form

$$\{X^j \in d\} \cup \{X^j \in \bar{d}\},$$

where d and $\bar{d}$ are not empty and define a partition of the finite set of possible values of the variable X^j.

Remark 2.1 In CART, we can take into account underrepresented classes by using prior probabilities. The relative probability assigned to each class can be used to adjust the magnitude of classification errors for each class. Another way of doing this is to oversample observations from rare classes, which is more or less equivalent to an overweighting of these observations.

Once the root of the tree has been split, we consider each of the child nodes and then, using the same procedure, we look for the best way to split them into two new nodes, and so on. The tree is thus developed until a stopping condition is reached. The most natural condition is not to split a pure node, i.e., a node containing only observations with the same outputs (typically in classification). But this criterion can lead to unnecessarily deep trees. It is often associated with the classical criterion of not splitting nodes that contain less than a given number of observations. The terminal nodes, which are no longer split, are called the leaves of the tree. We will

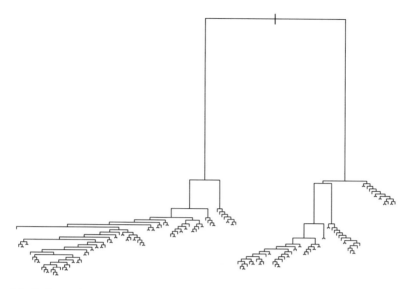

Fig. 2.3 Skeleton of the maximal tree, spam data

call the fully developed tree, the maximal tree, and denote it by $T_{\max}$. At the same time, each node t of the tree is associated with a value: $\overline{y}_t$ for regression or the label of the majority class of observations present in the node t in the classification case. Thus, a tree is associated not only with a partition defined by its leaves but also by the values that are attached to each piece of this partition. The tree predictor is then the piecewise constant function associated with the tree (Fig. 2.2).

The skeleton of the maximal tree on spam data is plotted in Fig. 2.3. Note that the edges are all not of the same length. In fact, the height of an edge connecting a node to its two children is proportional to the reduction in heterogeneity resulting from the splitting. Thus, for splits close to the root, the homogeneity gains are significant while for those located toward the leaves of the maximal tree, the gains are very small.

2.3 Pruning

Pruning is the second step of the CART algorithm. It consists in searching for the best pruned subtree of the maximal tree, the best in the sense of the generalization error. The idea is to look for a good intermediate tree between the two extremes: the maximal tree which has a high variance and a low bias, and the tree consisting only of the root (which corresponds to a constant predictor) which has a very low variance but a high bias. Pruning is a model selection procedure, where the competing models are the pruned subtrees of the maximal tree, i.e., all binary subtrees of $T_{\max}$ having the same root as $T_{\max}$.

Since the number of these subtrees is finite, it would therefore be possible, at least in principle, to build the sequence of all the best trees with k leaves for $1 \le k \le |T_{max}|$, where $|T|$ denotes the number of leaves of the tree T, and compare them, for example, on a test sample. However, the number of admissible models is exponential in the characteristic sizes of the learning data leading to an explosive algorithmic complexity. Fortunately, an effective alternative allows a sufficient implicit enumeration to achieve an optimal result. The process simply consists in the pruning algorithm, which ensures the extraction of a sequence of nested subtrees (i.e., pruned from each other) $T_1, \ldots, T_K$ all pruned from T_{max}, where T_k minimizes a penalized criterion where the penalty term is proportional to the number of leaves of the tree. This sequence is obtained iteratively by cutting branches at each step, which reduces complexity to a reasonable level. In the following few lines, we will limit ourselves to the regression case, the situation being identical in the classification case.

The key idea is to penalize the training error of a subtree T pruned from T_{max}

$$\overline{\text{err}}(T) = \frac{1}{n} \sum_{\{t \text{ leaf of } T\}} \sum_{(x_i, y_i) \in t} (y_i - \bar{y}_t)^2 \tag{2.1}$$

by a linear function of the number of leaves $|T|$ leading to the following penalized least squares criterion:

$$\text{crit}_\alpha(T) = \overline{\text{err}}(T) + \alpha|T| .$$

Thus, $\overline{\text{err}}(T)$ measures the fit of the model T to the data and decreases when the number of leaves increases while $|T|$ quantifies the complexity of the model T. The parameter α, positive, tunes the intensity of the penalty: the larger the coefficient α, the more penalized are the complex models, i.e., with many leaves.

The pruning algorithm is summarized in Table 2.1, with the following conventions. For any internal node (i.e., a node that is not a leaf) t of a tree T, we note T_t the branch of T resulting from the node t, i.e., all descendants of the node t. The error of the node t is given by $\overline{\text{err}}(t) = n^{-1} \sum_{\{x_i \in t\}} (y_i - \bar{y}_t)^2$ and the error of the tree T_t $\overline{\text{err}}(T_t)$ is defined by Eq. 2.1.

The central result of the book of Breiman et al. (1984) states that the strictly increasing sequence of parameters $(0 = \alpha_1, \ldots, \alpha_K)$ and the associated with the sequence $T_1 \succ \cdots \succ T_K$ made up of nested models (in the sense of pruning) are such for all $1 \le k \le K$:

$$\forall \alpha \in [\alpha_k, \alpha_{k+1}[\quad T_k = \underset{\{T \text{ subtree of } T_{max}\}}{\text{argmin}} \text{crit}_\alpha(T)$$

$$= \underset{\{T \text{ subtree of } T_{max}\}}{\text{argmin}} \text{crit}_{\alpha_k}(T)$$

by setting $\alpha_{K+1} = \infty$.

Table 2.1 CART pruning algorithm

Input	Maximal tree $T_{\max}$
Initialization	$\alpha_1 = 0, T_1 = T_{\alpha_1} = \operatorname{argmin}_T \text{ pruned from } T_{\max} \ \overline{\text{err}}(T).$
	initialize $T = T_1$ and $k = 1$
Iteration	While $\|T\| > 1$,
	Calculate
	$$\alpha_{k+1} = \min_{\{t \text{ internal node of } T\}} \frac{\overline{\text{err}}(t) - \overline{\text{err}}(T_t)}{\|T_t\| - 1}.$$
	Prune all T_t branches of T such that
	$$\overline{\text{err}}(T_t) + \alpha_{k+1}\|T_t\| = \overline{\text{err}}(t) + \alpha_{k+1}$$
	Take T_{k+1} the pruned subtree thus obtained
	Loop on $T = T_{k+1}$ et $k = k+1$
Output	Trees $T_1 \succ \cdots \succ T_K = \{t_1\}$,
	Parameters $(0 = \alpha_1; \ldots; \alpha_K)$

In other words, the sequence T_1 (which is nothing else than $T_{\max}$), $T_2, \ldots, T_K$ (which is nothing else than the tree reduced to the root) contains all the useful information since for any $\alpha \geqslant 0$, the subtree minimizing crit_α is a subtree of the sequence produced by the pruning algorithm.

This sequence can be visualized by means of the sequence of values $(\alpha_k)_{1 \leq k \leq K}$ and the generalization errors of the corresponding trees $T_1, \ldots, T_K$. In the graph of Fig. 2.5 obtained on the spam data (see p. 20), each point represents a tree: the abscissa is placed according to the value of the corresponding α_k, the ordinate according to the error estimated by cross-validation with the estimation of the standard deviation of the error materialized by a vertical segment.

The choice of the optimal tree can be made directly, by minimizing the error obtained by cross-validation or by applying the "1 standard error rule" ("1-SE rule" in brief). This rule aims at selecting in the sequence a more compact tree reaching statistically the same error. It consists in choosing the most compact tree reaching an error lower than the value of the previous minimum augmented by the estimated standard error of this error. This quantity is represented by the horizontal dotted line on the example of Fig. 2.5.

Remark 2.2 The cross-validation procedure (V-fold cross-validation), executed by default in the **rpart** package is as follows. First, starting from $\mathcal{L}_n$ and applying the pruning algorithm, we obtain the sequences $(T_k)_{1 \leq k \leq K}$ and $(\alpha_k)_{1 \leq k \leq K}$. Then, the learning sample is randomly divided into subsamples (often $V = 10$) so that $\mathcal{L}_n = E_1 \cup E_2 \cup \cdots \cup E_V$. For each $v = 1, \ldots, V$, we build the sequence of subtrees $(T_k^v)_{1 \leq k \leq K_v}$ with $\mathcal{L}_n \setminus E_v$ as learning sample. Then we calculate the validation errors of the sequence of trees built on $\mathcal{L}_n$: $R^{cv}(T_k) = \frac{1}{V} \sum_{v=1}^{V} \sum_{(x_i, y_i) \in E_v} \left(y_i - T_k^v(x_i) \right)^2$, where T_k^v minimizes the penalized criterion $\mathrm{crit}_{\alpha_k'}$, with $\alpha_k' = (\alpha_k \alpha_{k+1})^{1/2}$. We finally choose the model $T_{\hat{k}}$ where $\hat{k} = \mathrm{argmin}_{1 \leq k \leq K} R^{cv}(T_k)$.

Let us mention that the choice of α by a validation sample is not available in the **rpart** package.

Finally, it should be noted that, of course, if a tree in the sequence has k leaves, it is the best tree with k leaves. On the other hand, this sequence does not necessarily contain all the best trees with k leaves for $1 \leq k \leq |T_{\max}|$ but only a part of them. However, the "missing" trees are simply not competitive because they correspond to larger values of the penalized criterion, so it is useless to calculate them. In addition their calculation could be more expensive since they are not, in general, pruned from the trees of the sequence.

As we will see below, random forests are, in most cases, forests of unpruned trees. However, it should be stressed that a CART tree, if it used alone, must be pruned. Otherwise, it would suffer from overfitting by being too adapted to the data in $\mathcal{L}_n$ and exhibit a too large generalization error.

2.4 The rpart Package

The **rpart** package (Therneau and Atkinson 2018) implements the CART method as a whole and is installed by default in R. The `rpart()` function allows to build a tree whose development is controlled by the parameters of the `rpart.control()` function and pruning is achieved through the `prune()` function. Finally, the methods `print()`, `summary()`, `plot()`, and `predict()` allow retrieving and illustrate the results. It should also be noted that **rpart** fully handles missing data, both for prediction (see Sect. 2.5.2) and for learning (see details on the `Ozone` example in Sect. 2.6.1).

Other packages that implement decision trees are used in R, such as

- **tree** (Ripley 2018), quite close to **rpart** but which allows, for example, to trace the partition associated with a tree in small dimension and use a validation sample for pruning.
- **rpart.plot** (Milborrow 2018) which offers advanced graphics functions.
- **party** (Hothorn et al. 2017) which proposes other criteria for optimizing the splitting of a node.

Now let us detail the use of the functions `rpart()` and `prune()` on the spam detection example.

The tree built with the default values of `rpart()` is obtained as follows. Note that only the syntax `formula =`, `data =` is allowed for this function.

```
> library(rpart)
> treeDef <- rpart(type ~ ., data = spamApp)
> print(treeDef, digits = 2)
```

```
n= 2300

node), split, n, loss, yval, (yprob)
        * denotes terminal node

  1) root 2300 910 ok (0.606 0.394)
    2) charExclamation< 0.08 1369 230 ok (0.834 0.166)
      4) remove< 0.045 1263 140 ok (0.892 0.108)
        8) money< 0.15 1217 100 ok (0.917 0.083) *
        9) money>=0.15 46  11 spam (0.239 0.761) *
      5) remove>=0.045 106  15 spam (0.142 0.858) *
    3) charExclamation>=0.08 931 250 spam (0.271 0.729)
      6) charDollar< 0.0065 489 240 ok (0.489 0.511)
       12) capitalAve< 2.8 307 100 ok (0.674 0.326)
         24) remove< 0.09 265  60 ok (0.774 0.226)
           48) free< 0.2 223  31 ok (0.861 0.139) *
           49) free>=0.2 42  13 spam (0.310 0.690) *
         25) remove>=0.09 42   2 spam (0.048 0.952) *
       13) capitalAve>=2.8 182  32 spam (0.176 0.824)
         26) hp>=0.1 14   2 ok (0.857 0.143) *
         27) hp< 0.1 168  20 spam (0.119 0.881) *
      7) charDollar>=0.0065 442  13 spam (0.029 0.971) *
```

```
> plot(treeDef)
> text(treeDef, xpd = TRUE)
```

The `print()` method allows to obtain a text representation of the obtained decision tree, and the sequence of methods `plot()` then `text()` give a graphical representation (Fig. 2.4).

Remark 2.3 Caution, contrary to what one might think, the tree obtained with the default values of the package is not an optimal tree in the pruning sense. In fact, it is a tree whose development has been stopped, thanks to the parameters `minsplit` (the minimum number of data in a node necessary for the node to be possibly split) and `cp` (the normalized complexity-penalty parameter), documented in the `rpart.control()` function help page. Thus, as `cp = 0.01` by default, the tree provided corresponds to the one obtained by selecting the one corresponding to $\alpha = 0.01 * \overline{err}(T_n)$ (where T_1 is the root), provided that `minsplit` is not the parameter that stops the tree development. It is therefore not the optimal tree but generally a more compact one.

The maximal tree is then obtained using the following command (using the `set.seed()` function to ensure reproducibility of cross-validation results):

```
> set.seed(601334)
> treeMax <- rpart(type ~ ., data = spamApp, minsplit = 2, cp = 0)
> plot(treeMax)
```

The application of the `plot()` method allows to obtain the skeleton of the maximal tree (Fig. 2.3).

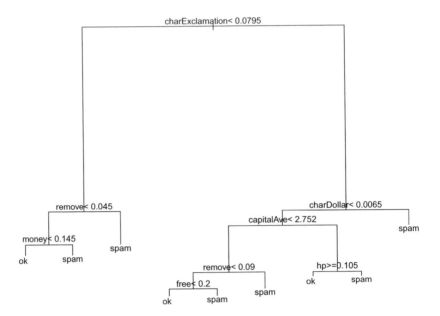

Fig. 2.4 Classification tree obtained with the default values of rpart(), spam data

Information on the optimal sequence of the pruned subtrees of $T_{\max}$ obtained by applying the pruning algorithm is given by the command:

```
> treeMax$cptable
```

In the columns of Table 2.2, we find the value of the penalty parameter, the number of splits of the corresponding optimal tree, the relative empirical error with respect to the one made by the tree restricted to the root, then the relative cross-validation error, and an estimate of the standard deviation of the associated estimator.

More graphically, we can visualize the sequence of the pruned subtrees of $T_{\max}$ (Fig. 2.5), thanks to the plotcp() function:

```
> plotcp(treeMax)
```

Each point thus represents a tree, with the estimation of the standard deviation of the cross-validation error as a vertical segment, quite hard to distinguish on this example (see Fig. 2.11 for a more meaningful graph). The position of the point indicates on the y-axis the (relative) cross-validation error, on the bottom x-axis the value of the penalty parameter, and on the top x-axis the number of leaves of the tree.

The shape of this graph is typical. Let us read it from left to right. When the model is too simple, the bias dominates and the error is significant. Then, it decreases fairly quickly until it reaches a minimum reflecting a good balance between bias and variance and finally rises slightly as the complexity of the model increases.

Table 2.2 Component `cptable` of the object `treeMax`, `spam` data

CP	nsplit	rel error	xerror	xstd
0.4713	0	1.0000	1.0000	0.0259
0.0839	1	0.5287	0.5519	0.0218
0.0591	2	0.4448	0.4570	0.0203
0.0419	4	0.3267	0.3565	0.0184
0.0265	5	0.2848	0.3146	0.0174
0.0177	6	0.2583	0.2947	0.0170
0.0110	7	0.2406	0.2815	0.0166
0.0088	8	0.2296	0.2638	0.0162
0.0055	9	0.2208	0.2517	0.0158
0.0044	14	0.1932	0.2483	0.0157
0.0039	16	0.1843	0.2528	0.0158
0.0033	18	0.1766	0.2373	0.0154
0.0028	24	0.1567	0.2296	0.0152
0.0022	26	0.1512	0.2296	0.0152
0.0015	48	0.1015	0.2307	0.0152
0.0015	53	0.0938	0.2329	0.0153
0.0011	56	0.0894	0.2351	0.0153
0.0009	102	0.0386	0.2439	0.0156
0.0008	110	0.0309	0.2506	0.0158
0.0007	118	0.0243	0.2494	0.0158
0.0006	124	0.0199	0.2517	0.0158
0.0006	131	0.0155	0.2704	0.0163
0.0004	153	0.0033	0.2726	0.0164
0.0000	162	0.0000	0.2759	0.0165

In addition, we find in Fig. 2.6 the same cross-validation error together with the empirical error. This last one decreases until reaching 0 for the maximal tree.

The tree minimizing the cross-validation error is sometimes still a little too complex (23 leaves here).

The optimal pruned tree is plotted in Fig. 2.7 and is obtained by

```
> cpOpt <- treeMax$cptable[which.min(treeMax$cptable[, 4]), 1]
> treeOpt <- prune(treeMax, cp = cpOpt)
> plot(treeOpt)
> text(treeOpt, xpd = TRUE, cex = 0.8)
```

By relaxing a little the condition of minimizing the generalization error by applying the "1-SE rule" of Breiman (which takes into account the uncertainty of the error estimation of the trees in the sequence), we obtain the tree of Fig. 2.8, the "1-SE" pruned tree:

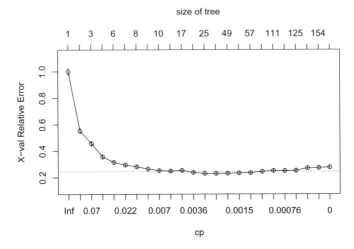

Fig. 2.5 Errors estimated by cross-validation of the sequence of subtrees pruned from the maximal tree, `spam` data

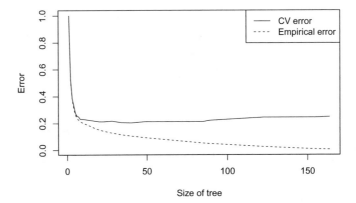

Fig. 2.6 Evolution of the error of pruned trees, learning and test, on the `spam` data

```
> thres1SE <- sum(treeMax$cptable[
    which.min(treeMax$cptable[, 4]), 4:5])
> cp1SE <- treeMax$cptable[
    min(which(treeMax$cptable[, 4] <= thres1SE)), 1]
> tree1SE <- prune(treeMax, cp = cp1SE)
> plot(tree1SE)
> text(tree1SE, xpd = TRUE, cex = 0.8)
```

The best pruned subtree of the maximal tree (up to one standard deviation according to "1-SE" rule) has 19 leaves and only 15 of the 57 initial variables are involved in the splits associated with the 18 internal nodes: charExclamation,

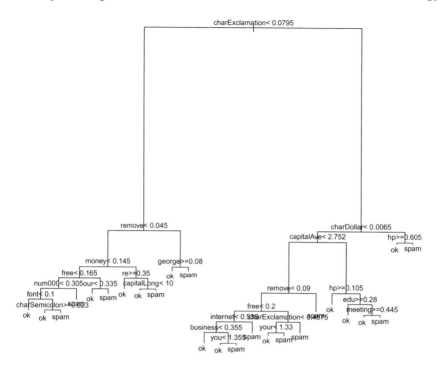

Fig. 2.7 Optimal pruned tree, spam data

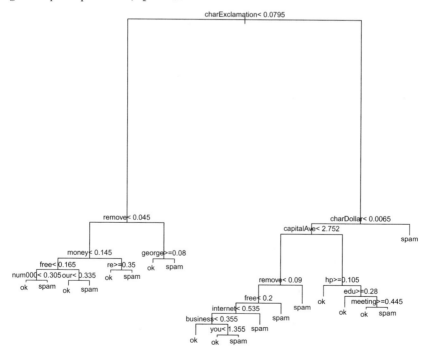

Fig. 2.8 Tree "1-SE" pruned, spam data

Table 2.3 Test and empirical errors for the maximal tree, optimal tree, 1-SE tree, and 2-leaf tree (Stump), spam data

	Max tree	Optimal tree	1-SE tree	Stump
Test error	0.096	0.086	0.094	0.209
Empirical error	0.000	0.062	0.070	0.208

charDollar, remove, capitalAve, money, george, hp, free, re, num000, our, edu, internet, business, and meeting.

We can illustrate the ease of interpretation by considering, for example, the path from the root to the rightmost leaf which says that an email containing a lot of "$" and "!" is almost always spam. Conversely, the path from the root to the third most right leaf expresses that an email containing a lot of "!", capital letters, and occurrences of the word hp but a few "$" is almost never spam. For this last interpretation, it is worth recalling that the emails examined are the professional emails of a single individual working for HP.

Finally, the empirical and test errors obtained by the different trees are summarized in Table 2.3 and calculated, for example, for the maximal tree, using the predict() function (which calculates the predictions for a given tree of a set of observations) by the following commands:

```
> errTestTreeMax <- mean(
    predict(treeMax, spamTest, type = "class") != spamTest$type)
> errEmpTreeMax <- mean(
    predict(treeMax, spamApp, type = "class") != spamApp$type)
```

It should be noted that, as announced, the maximal tree (too complex) has an empirical error (i.e., on the learning sample) of 0 and that the two-leaf tree (too simple) has similar test and empirical errors. The optimal tree has the best test error of 8.6%.

2.5 Competing and Surrogate Splits

2.5.1 Competing Splits

We have at each node of the tree, the sequence of all the splits (one per explanatory variable) ordered by decreasing reduction of the heterogeneity. These are called the competing splits. They are, in all nodes, necessarily calculated during the construction of the maximal tree but only a small number of them are, in general, kept (we refer to the summary of the object treeStump on the next page for an illustration on the spam data). The possibility of manual development of the maximal tree can be valuable and can be achieved by choosing in each of the nodes in the ordered list of splits, either the optimal one, or a slightly worse split. The actual split variable could be less uncertain, easier, cheaper to measure, or even more interpretable (see, for example, Ghattas 2000).

2.5.2 Surrogate Splits

One of the practical difficulties in calculating a prediction is the presence of missing values. CART offers an effective and very elegant way to circumvent it. First of all, it should be noted that when some input variables are missing for a given x, there is a problem only if the path to calculate the predicted value goes through a node whose split is based on one of these variables. Then, in a node where the split variable is missing, one of the other variables can be used, for example, the second competing split. But this idea is not optimal, since the routing rule in the right and left nodes, respectively, can be very different from the routing rule induced by the optimal split. Hence, the idea is to calculate at each node the list of surrogate splits, defined by the splits minimizing the number of routing errors with respect to the routing rule induced by the optimal split. This provides a method for handling missing values for prediction that is both local and efficient, avoiding to use global and often too coarse imputation methods.

These two aspects are illustrated by the following instructions.

```
> treeStump <- rpart(type ~ ., data = spamApp, maxdepth = 1)
> summary(treeStump)
```

```
Call:
rpart(formula = type ~ ., data = spamApp, maxdepth = 1)
  n= 2300


          CP nsplit rel error    xerror       xstd
1 0.4713024      0 1.0000000 1.0000000 0.02586446
2 0.0100000      1 0.5286976 0.5474614 0.02177043

Variable importance
charExclamation            free         your     charDollar
             44              12           12             12
      capitalLong             all
             11              10

Node number 1: 2300 observations,     complexity param=0.4713024
    predicted class=ok     expected loss=0.393913   P(node) =1
      class counts:   1394    906
     probabilities: 0.606 0.394
    left son=2 (1369 obs) right son=3 (931 obs)
    Primary splits:
```

```
           charExclamation < 0.0795 to the left,   improve=351.9304
           charDollar      < 0.0555 to the left,   improve=337.1138
           free            < 0.095  to the left,   improve=296.6714
           remove          < 0.01   to the left,   improve=290.1446
           your            < 0.605  to the left,   improve=272.6889
     Surrogate splits:
           free        < 0.135   to the left,  agree=0.710, adj=0.285
           your        < 0.755   to the left,  agree=0.703, adj=0.267
           charDollar  < 0.0555  to the left,  agree=0.702, adj=0.264
           capitalLong < 53.5    to the left,  agree=0.694, adj=0.245
           all         < 0.325   to the left,  agree=0.685, adj=0.221

  Node number 2: 1369 observations
    predicted class=ok      expected loss=0.1658145  P(node) =0.5952174
      class counts:   1142    227
    probabilities: 0.834 0.166

  Node number 3: 931 observations
    predicted class=spam  expected loss=0.2706767  P(node) =0.4047826
      class counts:    252    679
    probabilities: 0.271 0.729
```

This tree is the default tree of depth 1 (called *stump*), a typical weak classifier. The result of the method summary() provides information not only about the visible parts of the tree (such as structure and splits) but also about the hidden parts, involving variables that do not necessarily appear in the selected tree. Thus, we first find competing splits and then surrogate splits. It should be noted that to mimic the optimal routing rule, the best alternative split is free < 0.135 which differs from the competing split based on the same variable that is free < 0.095.

2.5.3 Interpretability

The interpretability of CART trees is one of the ingredients of their success. It is indeed very easy to answer the question of why, for a given x, a particular value of y is expected. To do this, it suffices to provide the sequence of the answers to the questions constituted by the successive splits encountered to go through the only path from the root to the associated leaf.

But more generally, beyond the interpretation of a particular prediction, once the CART tree has been built, we can consider the variables that intervene in the splits of the nodes of the tree. It is natural to think that the variables involved in splits close to the root are the most important, since they correspond to those whose contribution to the heterogeneity reduction is important. In a complementary way, we would tend to think that the variables that do not appear in any split are not important. Actually, this first intuition gives partial and biased results. Indeed, variables that do not appear in the tree can be important and even useful in this same model to deal with the problem of missing data in prediction, for example. A more sophisticated variable importance index is provided by CART trees. It is based on the concept of surrogate splits. According to Breiman et al. (1984), the importance of a variable can be defined by evaluating, in each node, the heterogeneity reduction generated by the use of the surrogate split for that variable and then summing them over all nodes.

In **rpart**, the importance of the variable X^j is defined by the sum of two terms. The first is the sum of the heterogeneity reductions generated by the splits involving X^j, and the second is weighted the sum of the heterogeneity reductions generated by the surrogate splits when X^j does not define the split. In the second case, the weighting is equal to the relative agreement, in excess of the majority routing rule, given for a node t of size n_t, by

$$\begin{cases} (n_{X^j} - n_{\mathrm{maj}})/(n_t - n_{\mathrm{maj}}) & \text{if } n_{X^j} > n_{\mathrm{maj}} \\ 0 & \text{otherwise} \end{cases}$$

where n_{X^j} and n_{maj} are the numbers of observations well routed with respect to the optimal split of the node t, respectively, by the surrogate split involving X^j and by the split according to the majority rule (which routes all observations to the child node of largest size). This weighting reflects the adjusted relative agreement between the optimal routing rule and the one associated with the surrogate split involving X^j, in excess of the majority rule. The raw relative agreement would be simply given by n_{X^j}/n_t.

However, as interesting as this variable importance index may be, it is no longer so widely used today. It is indeed not very intuitive, it is unstable because it is strongly dependent on a given tree, and it is less relevant than the importance of variables by permutation in the sense of random forests. In addition, its analog, which does not use surrogate splits, exists for random forests but tends to favor nominal variables that have a large number of possible values (we will come back to this in Sect. 4.1).

```
> par(mar = c(7, 3, 1, 1) + 0.1)
> barplot(treeMax$variable.importance, las = 2, cex.names = 0.8)
```

Nevertheless, it can be noted that the variable importance indices, in the sense of CART, for the maximal tree (given by Fig. 2.9) provide for the spam detection example very reasonable and easily interpretable results. It makes it possible to identify a group of variables: charExclamation clearly at the top then capitalLong, charDollar, free and remove then, less clearly, a group of 8 variables among which capitalAve, capitalTotal, money but also your and num000 intuitively less interesting.

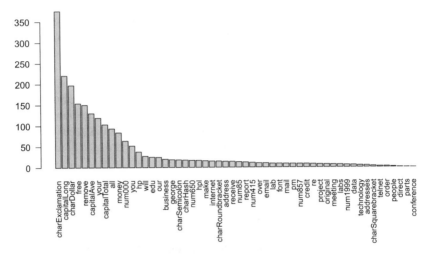

Fig. 2.9 Importance of variables in the sense of CART for the maximal tree, spam data

2.6 Examples

2.6.1 Predicting Ozone Concentration

For a presentation of this dataset, see Sect. 1.5.2.

Let us load the **rpart** package and the Ozone data:

```
> library("rpart")
> data("Ozone", package = "mlbench")
```

Let us start by building a tree using the default values of rpart():

```
> OzTreeDef <- rpart(V4 ~ ., data = Ozone)
> plot(OzTreeDef)
> text(OzTreeDef, xpd = TRUE, cex = 0.9)
```

Note that the response variable is in column 4 of the data Table and is denoted by V4.

Let us analyze this first tree (Fig. 2.10). This dataset has already been considered in many studies and, although these are real data, the results are relatively easy to interpret.

Looking at the first splits in the tree, we notice that the variables V8, V10 then V1 and V2 define them. Let us explain why.

Ozone is a secondary pollutant, since it is produced by the chemical transformation of primary precursor gases generated directly from the exhaust pipes (hydrocarbons and nitrogen oxides) in the presence of a catalyst for the chemical reaction: ultraviolet

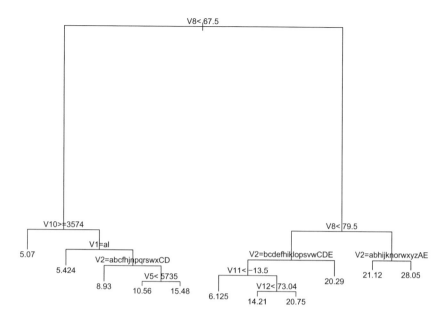

Fig. 2.10 Default tree, Ozone data

radiation. The latter is highly correlated with temperature (V8 or V9), which is one of the most important predictors of ozone. As a result, ozone concentrations peak during the summer months and this explains why the month number (V1) is among the influential variables. Finally, above an agglomeration, the pollutants are dispersed in a box whose base is the agglomeration and whose height is given by the inversion base height (V10).

Continuing to explore the tree, we notice that V2 defines splits quite close to the root of the tree, despite the fact that V2 is the number of the day within the month whose relationship with the response variable can only be caused by sampling effects. The explanation is classical in tree-based methods: it comes from the fact that V2 is a nominal variable with many possible values (here 31) involving a favorable selection bias when choosing the best split.

Predictions can also be easily interpreted: for example, the leftmost leaf gives very low predictions because it corresponds to cold days with a high inversion base height. On the other hand, the rightmost leaf provides much larger predictions because it corresponds to hot days.

Of course, it is now necessary to optimize the choice of the final tree. Let us study for that the sequence of the pruned subtrees (Fig. 2.11) which is the result of the pruning step starting from the the maximal tree.

```
> set.seed(727325)
> OzTreeMax <- rpart(V4 ~ ., data = Ozone, minsplit = 2, cp = 0)
> plotcp(OzTreeMax)
```

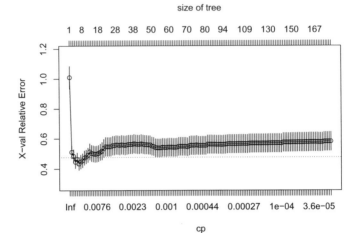

Fig. 2.11 Errors estimated by cross-validation of the sequence of subtrees pruned from the maximal tree, `Ozone` data

```
> OzIndcpOpt <- which.min(OzTreeMax$cptable[, 4])
> OzcpOpt <- OzTreeMax$cptable[OzIndcpOpt, 1]
> OzTreeOpt <- prune(OzTreeMax, cp = OzcpOpt)
> plot(OzTreeOpt)
> text(OzTreeOpt, xpd = TRUE)
```

The best tree (Fig. 2.12) is particularly compact since it has only six leaves, those involving splits on two of the three major variables highlighted above. We will see that a more complete, but above all, more automatic exploration of this aspect is provided by the permutation variable importance index in the context of random forests. This notion will allow eliminating the variable V2 whose interest is doubtful.

There is a lot of missing data in this dataset and `rpart()` offers a clever way to handle it during the learning step, without any imputation:

- The data with y missing are eliminated as well as those with all the components of x missing.
- Otherwise, to split a node:

  - Calculate the impurity reductions for each variable using only the associated available data and choose the best split as usual.
  - For this split, observations that have a missing value for the associated split variable are routed, either using a surrogate split or to the most popular node in case the variables determining the best available surrogate splits are all missing for this observation (the maximum number is a parameter, set to 5 by default).
  - Finally, weights in the impurity reduction are updated to take into account the new data routed.

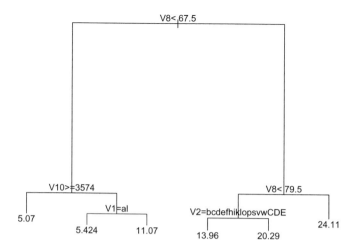

Fig. 2.12 Optimal pruned tree, `Ozone` data

2.6.2 Analyzing Genomic Data

For a presentation of this dataset, see Sect. 1.5.3.

Let us load the **rpart** package, the `vac18` data, and group in the same dataframe in which the gene expressions and the stimulation are to be predicted:

```
> library(rpart)
> data("vac18", package = "mixOmics")
> VAC18 <- data.frame(vac18$genes, stimu = vac18$stimulation)
```

The tree obtained with the default values of `rpart()` is obtained as follows (note the use of the argument `use.n = TRUE` in the `text()` function which displays the class distribution for each leaf):

```
> VacTreeDef <- rpart(stimu ~ ., data = VAC18)
> VacTreeDef
```

```
n= 42

node), split, n, loss, yval, (yprob)
      * denotes terminal node

1) root 42 31 LIPO5 (0.262 0.238 0.238 0.262)
  2) ILMN_2136089>=9.05 11  0 LIPO5 (1.000 0.000 0.000 0.000) *
  3) ILMN_2136089< 9.05 31 20 NS (0.000 0.323 0.323 0.355)
    6) ILMN_2102693< 8.59 18  8 GAG+ (0.000 0.556 0.444 0.000)*
    7) ILMN_2102693>=8.59 13  2 NS (0.000 0.000 0.154 0.846) *
```

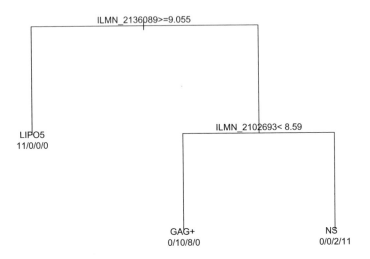

ILMN_2136089>=9.055

LIPO5
11/0/0/0

ILMN_2102693< 8.59

GAG+
0/10/8/0

NS
0/0/2/11

Fig. 2.13 Default tree obtained with `rpart()` on the `Vac18` data

```
> plot(VacTreeDef)
> text(VacTreeDef, use.n = TRUE, xpd = TRUE)
```

The default tree, represented in Fig. 2.13, consists of only 3 leaves. This is due, on the one hand, to the fact that there are only 42 observations in the dataset, and, on the other hand, that the classes LIPO5 and NS are separated from the others very quickly. Indeed, that the first split sends all the observations of class LIPO5, and only them, to the left child node.

The maximal tree has 6 leaves (Fig. 2.14). Thus in 5 splits, the classes are perfectly separated. We see on this example that considering only the variables appearing in the splits of a tree (here the deepest tree which can be built using these data) can be very restrictive: indeed, only 5 variables (corresponding to probe identifiers of biochips) among the 1,000 variables appear in the tree.

```
> set.seed(788182)
> VacTreeMax <- rpart(stimu ~ ., data = VAC18, minsplit = 2, cp = 0)
> plot(VacTreeMax)
> text(VacTreeMax, use.n = TRUE, xpd = TRUE)
```

The error estimated by validation for the sequence of pruned subtrees is plotted in the left graph of Fig. 2.15.

Given the small number of individuals, a leave-one-out estimate of the cross-validation error may be preferred. This is obtained by setting the argument `xval`, the number of folds of the cross-validation (argument of the `rpart.control()` function), as follows:

```
> set.seed(413745)
> VacTreeMaxLoo <- rpart(stimu ~ ., data = VAC18, minsplit = 2,
```

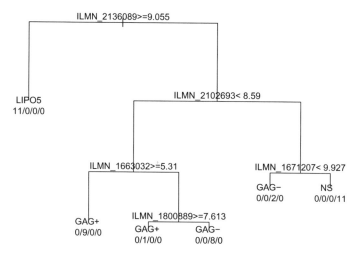

Fig. 2.14 Maximal tree on `Vac18` data

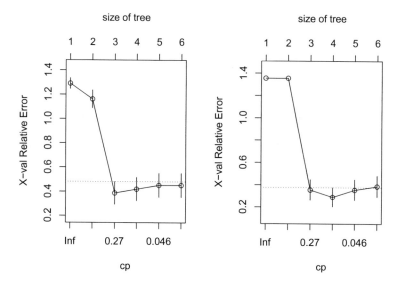

Fig. 2.15 Errors estimated by 10-fold cross-validation (left) and leave-one-out (right) of the sequence of subtrees pruned from the maximal tree, `Vac18` data

```
      cp = 0, xval = nrow(VAC18))
> par(mfrow = c(1, 2))
> plotcp(VacTreeMax)
> plotcp(VacTreeMaxLoo)
```

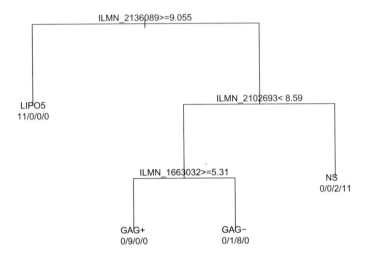

Fig. 2.16 Optimal pruned tree, `Vac18` data

We can easily see on the right side of Fig. 2.15 that for leave-one-out cross-validation, the optimal tree consists of 4 leaves while the 1-SE tree is the same as the default tree (3 leaves). The optimal tree (Fig. 2.16) is obtained using the following commands:

```
> VacIndcpOpt <- which.min(VacTreeMaxLoo$cptable[, 4])
> VaccpOpt <- VacTreeMaxLoo$cptable[VacIndcpOpt, 1]
> VacTreeOpt <- prune(VacTreeMaxLoo, cp = VaccpOpt)
> plot(VacTreeOpt)
> text(VacTreeOpt, use.n = TRUE, xpd = TRUE)
```

Chapter 3
Random Forests

Abstract The general principle of random forests is to aggregate a collection of random decision trees. The goal is, instead of seeking to optimize a predictor "at once" as for a CART tree, to pool a set of predictors (not necessarily optimal). Since individual trees are randomly perturbed, the forest benefits from a more extensive exploration of the space of all possible tree predictors, which, in practice, results in better predictive performance. Focusing on random forests, this chapter begins by addressing the instability of a tree and subsequently introduces readers to two random forest variants: Bagging and Random Forest Random Inputs. The construction of random forests is illustrated on the spam dataset using the randomForest package. The clever prediction error estimate Out-Of-Bag Error is also presented. In turn, the chapter assesses the sensitivity of prediction performance to the two main parameters: the number of trees and the number of variables picked at each node. In the final section, random forests are applied to three examples: predicting ozone concentration, analyzing genomic data, and analyzing dust pollution.

3.1 General Principle

The general principle of random forests (RF henceforth) is to aggregate a collection of random decision trees. The goal is, instead of seeking to optimize a predictor "at once" as for a CART tree, to pool a set of predictors (not necessarily optimal). Since · individual trees are randomly perturbed, the forest benefits from a more extensive exploration of the space of all possible tree predictors, which, in practice, results in better predictive performance.

The general definition of random forests, given by Breiman (2001), is as follows:

Definition 3.1 (*Random forests*) Let $\left(\widehat{h}(., \Theta_1), \ldots, \widehat{h}(., \Theta_q)\right)$ be a collection of tree predictors, with $\Theta_1, \ldots, \Theta_q$ q i.i.d. random variables independent of $\mathcal{L}_n$. The random forest predictor $\widehat{h}_{RF}$ is obtained by aggregating this collection of random trees. The aggregation is done as follows:

© Springer Nature Switzerland AG 2020
R. Genuer and J.-M. Poggi, *Random Forests with R*, Use R!,
https://doi.org/10.1007/978-3-030-56485-8_3

Fig. 3.1 General scheme of random forests

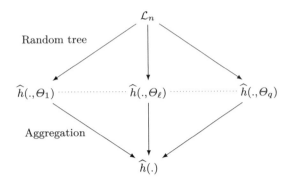

- $\widehat{h}_{RF}(x) = \dfrac{1}{q} \sum_{\ell=1}^{q} \widehat{h}(x, \Theta_\ell)$ (average of individual tree predictions) in regression.

- $\widehat{h}_{RF}(x) = \underset{1 \leq c \leq C}{\arg\max} \sum_{\ell=1}^{q} \mathbf{1}_{\widehat{h}(x,\Theta_\ell)=c}$ (majority vote among individual tree predictions) in classification.

Remark 3.1 Actually, this definition is not exactly the same as that of Breiman (2001), which does not specify that the variables Θ_ℓ are independent of $\mathcal{L}_n$. However, we adopt Definition 3.1 in this book because we find it more appropriate. Indeed, it is consistent with the intuition that the additional randomness provided by the Θ_ℓ is disconnected from the learning sample and, in addition, it encompasses the most commonly used RF variants.

This definition is illustrated by the diagram in Fig. 3.1. This scheme will be adapted several times later in this chapter, depending on the different RF methods presented.

In order to obtain good predictive performance, a random forest method must build a collection of trees that is

- As diverse as possible, because aggregating a set of predictors that are all very similar would give nothing more than again a similar predictor.
- Made up of individual predictors with acceptable predictive capacity, because if for a new observation x all trees provide a bad prediction, the aggregation of these predictions has no chance of being correct.

3.1.1 Instability of a Tree

Before presenting different RF variants, we illustrate a well-known property of CART trees, namely their instability. Instability here means that if the learning sample on which a CART tree is built is slightly modified, then the resulting tree is usually very different from the original tree.

To illustrate this behavior, let us build two CART trees (with parameter default values of the `rpart()` function) from two different bootstrap samples, named `spamBoot1` and `spamBoot2`, derived from the `spam` data learning sample, `spamApp`. The notion of bootstrap samples is introduced in the following definition.

Definition 3.2 (*Bootstrap sample*) A bootstrap sample of a learning sample $\mathcal{L}_n$ of size n is obtained by randomly drawing n observations from $\mathcal{L}_n$ with replacement, each observation (X_i, Y_i) of $\mathcal{L}_n$ having a probability $1/n$ of being selected in each draw.

```
> set.seed(368910)
> spamBoot1 <- spamApp[
    sample(1:nrow(spamApp), nrow(spamApp), replace = TRUE), ]
> treeBoot1 <- rpart(type ~ ., data = spamBoot1)
> plot(treeBoot1)
> text(treeBoot1, xpd = TRUE)
```

```
> set.seed(368915)
> spamBoot2 <- spamApp[
    sample(1:nrow(spamApp), nrow(spamApp), replace = TRUE), ]
> treeBoot2 <- rpart(type ~ ., data = spamBoot2)
> plot(treeBoot2)
> text(treeBoot2, xpd = TRUE)
```

We note that the structures of the two trees (Figs. 3.2 and 3.3) are very different. This major difference is explained by the fact that, as illustrated, there are changes from the first splits (at the top of the tree). Thus, the recursive nature of CART tree building implies that these changes are reflected throughout the tree development. In addition, since the pruning step is conditional on the maximal tree, the differences observed would be as important for pruned trees.

If we compare them with the tree obtained in Fig. 2.4, we notice that the tree built on the sample `spamBoot2` is relatively similar to the one built on the whole learning sample `spamApp`. Thus, depending on the bootstrap sample, resulting trees could be very different from each other.

Finally, we could expect to see the variable `charDollar` appear in the root node split in such a situation, because in Sect. 2.5 we saw that it occurred in the first concurrent split of this node, with a value of `improve` relatively close to that of the original split (made on the variable `charExclamation`).

Now let us compare predictions given by the two previous trees on the test sample.

```
> mean(predict(treeBoot1, spamTest, type = "class") !=
    predict(treeBoot2, spamTest, type = "class"))
```

```
[1] 0.08822251
```

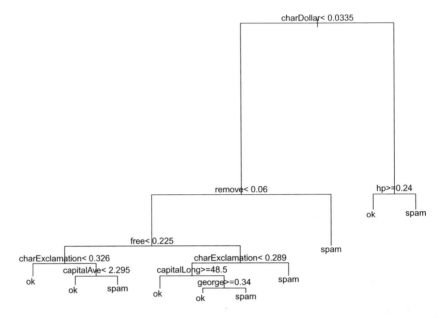

Fig. 3.2 Classification tree obtained with the default values of `rpart()` on the bootstrap sample `spamBoot1`; spam data

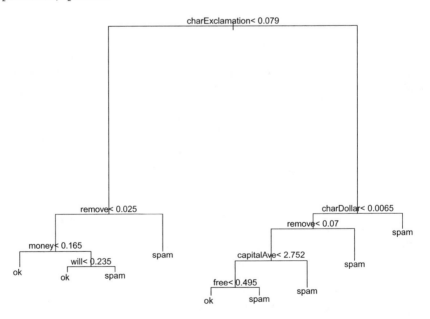

Fig. 3.3 Classification tree obtained with the default values of `rpart()` on the bootstrap sample `spamBoot2`, spam data

This result illustrates that the instability of CART trees also results in a variation of predictions. In our example, about 8.8% of the test data has an altered prediction.

3.1.2 From a Tree to an Ensemble: Bagging

The first historical example of a random forest method that verifies the conditions of Definition 3.1 is the Bagging method introduced by Breiman (1996). The word Bagging is the acronym for "**B**ootstrap **agg**regat**ing**". Thus, the Bagging predictor is obtained by aggregating a set of tree predictors, each constructed on a different bootstrap sample. This method is therefore a random forest where the hazard comes from the bootstrap draw.

The diagram of Fig. 3.4 summarizes the principle of Bagging.

To illustrate Bagging on spam data, we can use the **randomForest** package, presented in detail in Sect. 3.3.

The Bagging predictor is obtained using the following command, for which the mtry parameter of the randomForest() function is set to p, the number of explanatory variables, while all other parameters are kept to their default values. We will come back to the meaning of the mtry parameter in Sect. 3.2.

```
> library(randomForest)
> bagging <- randomForest(type ~ ., data = spamApp,
    mtry = ncol(spamApp) - 1)
> bagging
```

```
Call:
```

Fig. 3.4 Bagging diagram

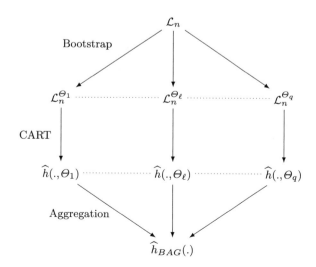

```
randomForest(formula = type ~ ., data = spamApp,
     mtry = ncol(spamApp) - 1)
                    Type of random forest: classification
                          Number of trees: 500
No. of variables tried at each split: 57

        OOB estimate of  error rate: 6.13%
Confusion matrix:
        ok spam class.error
ok    1339   55  0.03945481
spam    86  820  0.09492274
```

By default, 500 bootstrap samples are generated and a collection of 500 trees is therefore built before being aggregated.

Remark 3.2 The predictor thus created is not exactly Bagging, as defined in Fig. 3.4, because in fact maximal trees are built (and not optimal pruned trees as in CART). So we are considering here the maximal trees' Bagging instead. To our knowledge, the Bagging method with optimal pruned trees is not implemented directly in R. More specifically, in

- **ipred** (Peters and Hothorn 2017), all trees in Bagging can be pruned uniformly using the parameters of the `rpart.control()` function (see Sect. 2.4).
- **adabag** (Alfaro et al. 2013), the same uniform pruning can be obtained, but in addition, the `autoprune()` function which automatically calculates the optimal pruned tree can easily be used to code the optimal trees' Bagging.

Let us compute the test and learning errors obtained by Bagging on `spam` data using the `predict()` function (which calculates the predictions of a set of observations) and compare them to the errors obtained with CART trees (Table 3.1):

```
> errTestBagging <- mean(
    predict(bagging, spamTest) != spamTest$type)
> errEmpBagging <- mean(
    predict(bagging, spamApp) != spamApp$type)
```

In this example, the test error reached by Bagging is indeed lower than those obtained by the CART trees (only the smallest error, reached by the optimal tree and computed in Sect. 2.3, is recalled in the table). Intuitively, this decrease in prediction

Table 3.1 Test and empirical errors of the optimal tree and bagging, spam data

	Optimal tree	Bagging
Test error	0.086	0.062
Empirical error	0.062	0.000

error is due to CART instability. In fact, the instability of CART allows to build a set of trees relatively different from each other in Bagging, because they are built on different bootstrap samples.

In addition, Bagging, through aggregation, stabilizes CART trees. Indeed, by averaging (or applying the majority vote rule in classification) the individual trees, which are very different from each other, Bagging provides a stable predictor.

Remark 3.3 The Bagging method is very general, and could be used with any basic predictor, but the fact that it has been used most often with trees (or what are called weak predictors) comes precisely from the unstable nature of the latter. In other words, applying a Bagging method with a stable base predictor (such as logistic regression for spam data) does not bring any significant improvement.

3.2 Random Forest Random Inputs

Many RF methods, i.e., many types of additional hazards (the Θ_ℓ in Definition 3.1), have been tried since the late 1990s (Ho 1998; Dietterich 2000; Breiman 2000). However, one of them has become the reference method: it is the Random Forests-Random Inputs (RF-RI) algorithm, introduced by Breiman (2001). We now detail this variant, which we will call RF later on.

Remark 3.4 The language abuse consisting in naming the RF-RI method by RF is widely used in the literature on random forests. Indeed, very often we speak of random forests to designate this particular case of the much more general Definition 3.1.

"Random Inputs" must be understood here as "random input variables". The principle of RF-RI is then to aggregate a collection of tree predictors with random input variables, which we will call "RI trees", each built on a bootstrap sample (see Definition 3.2).

Definition 3.3 (*RI Tree*) An RI tree is a tree predictor, with the following major differences with a CART tree:

- At each node of a tree, we randomly select a subset of mtry variables, then we look for the best way to split this node only among the splits that involve these variables.
- Trees are not pruned.

The random selection of variables is done by a uniform draw of mtry variables without replacement among the p available variables.

A summary diagram of the RF-RI algorithm, where Θ refers to the bootstrap draw and Θ' refers to the random draw of variables can be found in Fig. 3.5.

Fig. 3.5 RF-RI random
forest scheme

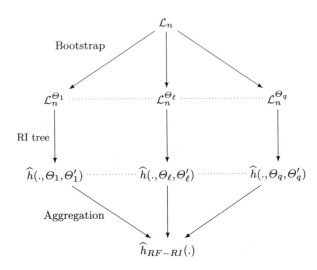

The general idea of this method is that the random perturbation on individuals, brought by bootstrap sample draws, is not sufficient to promote diversity among trees and that it is also necessary to perturb the construction of trees at the variable level. This perturbation is applied before optimal splitting search at each node. Thus, thanks to this additional randomness, an even more diversified collection of trees is built, which, in practice, leads to an additional improvement in predictive performance compared to Bagging.

Remark 3.5 It is important to note that the number of randomly selected variables, noted m**try** (for "number of variables tried to split a node"), is the most important parameter of the method, and that it is the same for all nodes of all trees in the forest.

In the spam example, we obtain a test error rate of 0.052 for an RF with default values for all parameters, which illustrates an improvement made by RF compared to Bagging and therefore to CART trees (Table 3.2).

Table 3.2 Test and empirical errors of the optimal tree, bagging, and RF spam data

	Optimal tree	Bagging	RF
Test error	0.086	0.062	0.052
Empirical error	0.062	0.000	0.004

3.3 The randomForest Package

The **randomForest** package was brought into R by Liaw and Wiener (2002) and is based on the initial Fortran code of Breiman and Cutler.[1] The source code of the package is structured in a rather complex way, with main functions in R that call C code, which itself calls Fortran code. However for the user, the package is very accomplished with a well-documented main function `randomForest()`, with usual R methods such as `print()`, `plot()`, `predict()` (no `summary()` method implemented) and other related functions that help to use or interpret random forests such as `importance()` (see Chap. 4) or `partialPlot()` (see Sect. 3.6.3).

Other R packages that implement random forests:

- **ranger** (Wright 2017) is optimized in C and is a very interesting alternative, especially when processing high-dimensional datasets. It often allows a significant reduction in computation times while providing essentially the same results as **randomForest**.
- **Rborist** (Seligman 2017) has an implementation dedicated to scale in the context of Big Data, where the number of observations n is very high;
- **party** (Hothorn et al. 2017) proposes a unified implementation of CART trees and random forest methods through the functions `ctree()` and `cforest()`.

Let us now detail the use of the `randomForest()` function which implements the RF-RI method. The main parameters of this function are

- `mtry`: the number of variables randomly selected at each node, which by default is $\sqrt{p}$ in classification and $p/3$ in regression (where p refers to the number of input variables).
- `ntree`: the number of trees in the forest, denoted as q in this chapter, which by default is 500.
- `nodesize`: the minimum number of observations that a leaf of a tree must contain, which by default is 1 in classification and 5 in regression.

Thus, to obtain an RF-RI predictor, trained on `spam` data, made of 500 trees and where the number of variables randomly drawn at each node is 7 (the integer part of $\sqrt{57}$), we use the following command:

```
> RFDef <- randomForest(type ~ ., data = spamApp)
> RFDef
```

```
Call:
 randomForest(formula = type ~ ., data = spamApp)
               Type of random forest: classification
```

---

[1] http://www.stat.berkeley.edu/~breiman/RandomForests/cc_manual.htm.

```
                     Number of trees: 500
  No. of variables tried at each split: 7

        OOB estimate of  error rate: 5.7%
Confusion matrix:
        ok spam class.error
ok    1344   50  0.03586801
spam    81  825  0.08940397
```

Unlike `rpart()` which only accepts calls of type "`formula =, data = `", `randomForest()` has an alternative syntax of type "`x = , y = `". Thus the following command is equivalent to the previous one (and is recommended for the application of `randomForest()` in high-dimensional cases, see Sect. 3.6.2):

```
> RFDef <- randomForest(spamApp[, -58], spamApp[, 58])
```

The empirical error and test rates contained in Table 3.2 are obtained using the `predict()` function (which computes the predictions of a set of observations) by the following commands:

```
> errTestRFDef <- mean(predict(RFDef, spamTest) != spamTest$type)
> errEmpRFDef <- mean(predict(RFDef, spamApp) != spamApp$type)
```

Remark 3.6 In Chen et al. (2004) are studied two ways to take into account unbalanced data using RF: Weighted RF that consists of putting more weight on the minority class, thus penalizing more heavily the classification errors of the minority class; Balanced RF that artificially modifies the distribution of classes so that they are represented more or less equally in each tree. The two variants can be easily implemented using `randomForest()` parameters: the `classwt` parameter for the priors (*a priori* probabilities) of the classes and the `strata` parameter for the stratified sampling of each bootstrap sample.

3.4 Out-Of-Bag Error

As we can see in the `RFDef` object print (see previous section), we have a direct estimate of the prediction error from the output of the `randomForest()` function. This estimate is of the same type as cross-validation and avoids the need for a test sample. It is called "OOB error", where "OOB" means "**O**ut **O**f **B**ag", and must be understood as "out of the Bootstrap". The main idea of this error estimator is to use observations that were not selected in a bootstrap sample as test data.[2] The exact definition is as follows.

---

[2]Bootstrapping leads on average to 37% of the observations out of the bootstrap sample.

Definition 3.4 (*OOB error*) To predict the ith observation X_i, we only aggregate predictors built on bootstrap samples *not containing* (X_i, Y_i). This provides a prediction $\widehat{Y}_i$ for the output of the ith observation.

The OOB error is then calculated as follows:

- $\frac{1}{n} \sum_{i=1}^{n} \left(Y_i - \widehat{Y}_i\right)^2$ in regression.
- $\frac{1}{n} \sum_{i=1}^{n} \mathbf{1}_{Y_i \neq \widehat{Y}_i}$ in classification.

This estimate is very often reasonable (for our two previous examples, Bagging and RF by default, it gives error rates very close to the test error), and can in any case be used to optimize RF parameters.

3.5 Parameters Setting for Prediction

3.5.1 The Number of Trees: `ntree`

The `ntree` parameter is not the most crucial one for the RF-RI method since the larger the number of trees, the better. The number of trees is therefore adjusted according to the forest's computation time and is large enough as soon as the addition of new trees to the forest does not bring any improvement in terms of prediction.

The `plot()` method implemented in the **randomForest** package plots the OOB error as a function of the number of trees in the forest (once the forest is built):

```
> plot(RFDef)
```

We see (Fig. 3.6) that the OOB error variations are very small as soon as the number of trees is large enough (for our example, from 100 trees the error stabilizes), and the default value (500) is here large enough.

Finally, let us note the existence of the `do.trace` option which can be useful to follow the evolution of the OOB error according to the number of trees during the construction of the forest itself:

```
> RFDoTrace <- randomForest(type ~ ., data = spamApp, ntree = 250,
    do.trace = 25)
```

```
ntree        OOB      1       2
  25:       6.30%  4.09%   9.71%
  50:       5.83%  3.59%   9.27%
  75:       5.48%  3.44%   8.61%
 100:       5.48%  3.23%   8.94%
 125:       5.61%  3.52%   8.83%
 150:       5.26%  3.52%   7.95%
 175:       5.57%  3.52%   8.72%
```

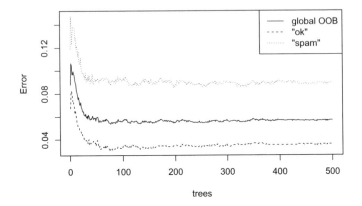

Fig. 3.6 Evolution of the global OOB error and for each class, according to the number of trees, spam data

```
200:    5.48%   3.23%   8.94%
225:    5.39%   3.30%   8.61%
250:    5.30%   3.16%   8.61%
```

3.5.2   The Number of Variables Chosen at Each Node: `mtry`

The `mtry` parameter is the most important parameter of the `randomForest()` function. Indeed, different values of this parameter can lead to very different predictive performance. Moreover, the optimal value of `mtry` will depend greatly on the total number of variables p (and also on the number of variables really related to Y, but the latter is unknown).

Since the total number of variables is not very large for spam data, we can try all possible values for `mtry` (i.e., all integers between 1 and p):

```
> nbvars <- 1:(ncol(spamApp) - 1)
> oobsMtry <- sapply(nbvars, function(nbv) {
    RF <- randomForest(type ~ ., spamApp, ntree = 250, mtry = nbv)
    return(RF$err.rate[RF$ntree, "OOB"])
  })
```

We can even stabilize the OOB error estimate by calculating an average of errors over several runs of `randomForest()`. For example, the following command calculates the average OOB error over 25 forests of 250 trees with the default value of `mtry`:

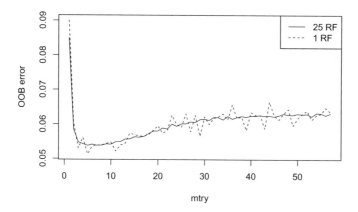

Fig. 3.7   OOB error as a function of `mtry` parameter value, `spam` data

```
> mean(replicate(n = 25, randomForest(type ~ ., spamApp,
    ntree = 250)$err.rate[250, "OOB"]))
```

The OOB error evolution (Fig. 3.7) according to `mtry` value on our `spam` example is typical of standard (i.e., not high-dimensional) classification problems:

- If `mtry` is really too low, then the OOB error is relatively high (the extreme case where `mtry` is 1 is to choose the split variable completely at random at each node).
- When we increase `mtry` the error decreases quickly, until it reaches a minimum, then the error rises gradually.

In regression, we observe most of the time a decreasing behavior of the OOB error as a function of `mtry`. The default value of the parameter is also higher in regression, equal to $p/3$ (instead of $\sqrt{p}$ in classification).

For a more detailed study of the `mtry` setting, we refer to Sect. 2 of Genuer et al. (2008).

Tree Diversity Illustration

To conclude this section, let us illustrate the notion of tree diversity in a simple case where only two-leaf trees (also called stumps) are considered. Let us start by building a Bagging predictor made of 100 stumps:

```
> bagStump <- randomForest(type ~ ., spamApp, ntree = 100,
    mtry = ncol(spamApp) - 1, maxnodes = 2)
```

Let us now look at which variables were used to split the root node of the 100 trees:

```
> bagStumpbestvar <- table(bagStump$forest$bestvar[1, ])
> names(bagStumpbestvar) <- colnames(spamApp)[
    as.numeric(names(bagStumpbestvar))]
> sort(bagStumpbestvar, decreasing = TRUE)
```

charExclamation	charDollar	free
70	29	1

We notice that the root node is (among the 100 trees) almost always split either with the charExclamation variable or the charDollar variable.

If we now consider an RF made of 100 stumps with the default value of mtry, i.e., 7:

```
> RFStump <- randomForest(type ~ ., spamApp, ntree = 100,
    maxnodes = 2)
> RFStumpbestvar <- table(RFStump$forest$bestvar[1, ])
> names(RFStumpbestvar) <- colnames(spamApp)[
    as.numeric(names(RFStumpbestvar))]
> sort(RFStumpbestvar, decreasing = TRUE)
```

free	charDollar	charExclamation	remove
12	12	11	9
your	capitalAve	num000	money
9	9	6	6
our	receive	you	credit
4	4	3	3
hp	capitalLong	address	business
3	3	2	1
hpl	george	capitalTotal	
1	1	1	

We see that the "diversity" of the splitting variables of the trees' root nodes is much larger. The charExclamation and charDollar variables are still among the most frequently chosen, but other variables were optimal for splitting, when charExclamation and charDollar did not belong to the selected variable set.

Even if this study is somewhat reductive because we limit ourselves only to what happens for the root node, it gives an idea of the increase in diversity brought by RF-RI compared to Bagging.

3.6 Examples

3.6.1 Predicting Ozone Concentration

For a presentation of this dataset, see Sect. 1.5.2.

Let us load the **randomForest** package and `Ozone` data:

```
> library("randomForest")
> data("Ozone", package = "mlbench")
```

Remark 3.7 It should be noted that, in this example, the standard theoretical framework that assumes observations as independent realizations from the same distribution is inappropriate. Indeed, the serial dependence between two successive observations is obvious and important since it carries both short-range dependence (the weather of the day is generally close to that of the next day) and long-range dependence because of the seasonal nature of both the weather and social life. Nevertheless, it appears that even in this context, random forests perform well.

Application of RF on this dataset can be done using the following command:

```
> OzRFDef <- randomForest(V4 ~ ., Ozone, na.action = na.omit)
```

Note that the response variable, named `V4`, is located in the 4th column of the data table. In addition, we must set the `na.action` parameter because we are dealing with missing data. It should be noted that there are many of them (about 45% of the observations contain at least one missing data) mainly because of `V9`. However, we will simply omit them here.

Remark 3.8 The `rfImpute()` function of the **randomForest** package allows to impute missing values using the proximities between complete observations. Proximity between two observations is the proportion of trees in which they appear in the same terminal node of a given forest. The iterative imputation procedure can be deduced from this: the first forest is built using the median imputation, the proximities are then calculated and new imputations are made by a weighted average according to the regression proximities or a weighted vote according to the classification proximities. A new forest is then built, giving new proximities and imputations, and the procedure is iterated until the last imputation.

Let us display the results of this random forest:

```
> OzRFDef
```

```
Call:
 randomForest(formula = V4 ~ ., data = Ozone, na.action = na.omit)
               Type of random forest: regression
                     Number of trees: 500
```

```
No. of variables tried at each split: 4

      Mean of squared residuals: 21.20203
                  % Var explained: 68.24
```

> **plot**(OzRFDef)

The plot of Fig. 3.8 illustrates both the gain brought by the aggregation of predictions provided by more and more trees (note, however, that compared to CART, the error of a single tree is increased here because the trees are not pruned) and the fact that increasing the number of trees no longer provides anything essential (at least for average performance) from 50 or 100 trees and nothing at all from 200 trees.

More interestingly, it illustrates the absence of overfitting. Indeed, despite the small number of observations (less than 400 and even 200 without missing values) compared to the maximum number of trees in the forest (here 500), there is no overfitting phenomenon: the error no longer decreases but does not increase either, it stabilizes.

In this example, the OOB error increases with `mtry` (Fig. 3.9), which is rather unusual. In this case, it can be explained by the importance of the variables (see Sect. 4.5.2).

Remark 3.9 In this example, the response variable distribution is very asymmetric and large ozone concentration values are rare. One way to take this aspect into account to some extent is to consider a stratified sampling, with respect to the concentration of pollutants (V4), when selecting OOB samples, so as to preserve the distribution of the response variable in both bootstrap and OOB samples.

Bootstrap samples, and consequently OOB samples, can be stratified by creating a factor, whose distribution will be used to stratify. Thus, we begin by dividing

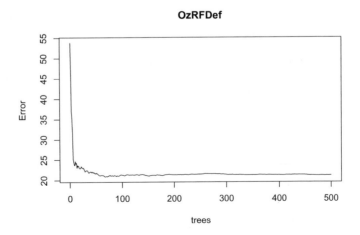

Fig. 3.8 OOB error as a function of the number of trees, Ozone data

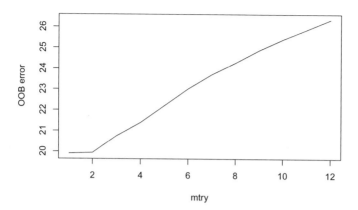

Fig. 3.9 OOB error as a function of `mtry` parameter value, `Ozone` data

the range of the response variable into 3 classes (values less than 10, between 10 and 20, and greater than 20) according to which the stratification is performed. The commands below show how to proceed while eliminating the second temperature variable that has a lot of missing data.

```
> bins <- c(0, 10, 20, 40)
> V4bin <- cut(Ozone$V4, bins, include.lowest = TRUE, right = FALSE)
> OzoneBin <- data.frame(Ozone, V4bin)
> OzRFDefStrat <- randomForest(V4 ~ . - V9 - V4bin, OzoneBin,
    strata = V4bin, sampsize = 200, na.action = na.omit)
> OzRFDefStrat
```

```
Call:
 randomForest(formula = V4 ~ . - V9 - V4bin, data = OzoneBin,
      strata = V4bin, sampsize = 200, na.action = na.omit)
               Type of random forest: regression
                     Number of trees: 500
No. of variables tried at each split: 3

        Mean of squared residuals: 22.22533
                  % Var explained: 66.7
```

The impact is not massive on this example, but in the case of ozone measured in cities with more pronounced seasonal contrasts, this type of stratification can be useful. In the following, we return to the basic version.

3.6.2 Analyzing Genomic Data

For a presentation of this dataset, see Sect. 1.5.3.

Let us load the **randomForest** package and vac18 data:

```
> library(randomForest)
> data("vac18", package = "mixOmics")
```

Then let us create an object geneExpr containing the gene expressions and an object stimu containing the stimuli to be predicted:

```
> geneExpr <- vac18$genes
> stimu <- vac18$stimulation
```

The training of a random forest is done with the following commands. Dealing with high-dimensional data, we set the value from mtry to $p/3$. We recommend this value of mtry in this case because the default value $\sqrt{p}$ (i.e., 31 in this example) generally leads to consider too few informative variables in each node (Fig. 3.11).

```
> VacRFpsur3 <- randomForest(x = geneExpr, y = stimu,
    mtry = ncol(geneExpr)/3)
> VacRFpsur3
> plot(VacRFpsur3)
```

```
Call:
 randomForest(x = geneExpr, y = stimu, mtry = ncol(geneExpr)/3)
               Type of random forest: classification
                     Number of trees: 500
No. of variables tried at each split: 333

        OOB estimate of  error rate: 35.71%
Confusion matrix:
      LIPO5 GAG+ GAG- NS class.error
LIPO5    11    0    0  0   0.0000000
GAG+      0    5    3  2   0.5000000
GAG-      0    4    2  4   0.8000000
NS        0    0    2  9   0.1818182
```

We see, thanks to the confusion matrix, giving in line the predicted class and in column the actual class, that the relatively high OOB error is largely due to the GAG– class which is predicted either in GAG+ or in NS. This is because the GAG– stimulation is not only quite close to a "non-stimulation" but also has common features with the GAG+ stimulation.

According to Fig. 3.10, the OOB error stabilizes after about 100 trees have been built.

VacRFpsur3

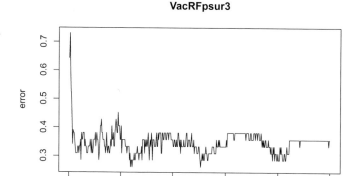

Fig. 3.10 OOB error evolution according to the number of trees in the forest (OOB errors per class have been hidden to facilitate the reading of the graph), Vac18 data

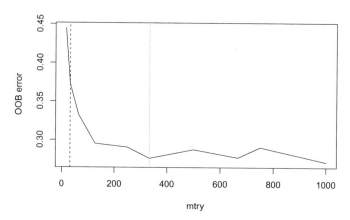

Fig. 3.11 OOB error evolution (averaged over 25 forests) as a function of the value of mtry, Vac18 data. The vertical dotted line indicates the value $p/3$, while the dashed line indicates the default value of mtry $\sqrt{p}$

In addition, we see that the OOB error is (roughly) decreasing when the value of mtry increases (Fig. 3.11) and stabilizes when mtry reaches $p/3$ in this example.

Computation time

We used the default syntax of randomForest() of the type "x = , y = ". In general, we prefer this syntax to the alternative syntax of the type "formula = , data = " because the first is by our experience often faster than the second when we apply RF to high-dimensional data.

Table 3.3 Comparison of execution times (medians on 25 runs) of the functions `randomForest()` and `ranger()`, Vac18 data

Function	Type	Time (in s)
randomForest()	formula	0.705
randomForest()	x, y	0.498
ranger()	formula	0.402
ranger()	x, y	0.392

Finally, still in the context of high-dimensional data, the use of the **ranger** package could give interesting results in terms of computation time (and according to our tests, the larger the dimension, the greater the gain).

A comparison of the computation times leads to the results of Table 3.3 (the times displayed are median execution times over 25 runs).

Finally, it should be noted that the `ranger()` function allows parallel computing natively. To do this, simply set the value of the `num.threads` parameter, which by default is set to the number of cores available on the computer running the code (we set it to 1 to compare only non-parallelized commands).

3.6.3   Analyzing Dust Pollution

For a presentation of this dataset, see Sect. 1.5.4.

Let us load the **randomForest** package and the JUS station data, included in the **VSURF package** and create a dataframe `jusComp` containing no missing data:

```
> library(randomForest)
> data("jus", package = "VSURF")
> jusComp <- na.omit(jus)
```

Random forests and partial effects
Random forests are a powerful and convenient tool to visualize, for each station, the effects of variables on PM10 pollution and to identify important variables among pollutants and weather variables.

```
> jusRF <- randomForest(PM10 ~ ., data = jusComp)
```

To estimate the marginal effect of variable X^j, we mimic the partial integration of the forest (i.e., the estimated regression function), by using an empirical mean which approximates the expectation according to all variables except X^j:

$$\tilde{f}_j(x) = \frac{1}{n} \sum_{i=1}^{n} \widehat{h}_{RF}(x_i^1, \ldots, x_i^{j-1}, x, x_i^{j+1}, \ldots, x_i^p) \, .$$

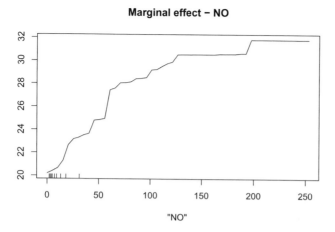

Fig. 3.12 Marginal effect of NO variable on PM10 concentration, associated with a random forest trained using station JUS data

The following command is used to compute the marginal effect of NO variable, at the JUS station (Fig. 3.12). In the same way, we can obtain marginal effects of all variables at the JUS station (Fig. 3.13).

```
> partialPlot(jusRF, pred.data = jusComp, x.var = "NO",
    main = "Marginal effect - NO")
```

Remark 3.10 To go further on partial effects study, and especially if we are interested in the effect of a pair of variables, we can use the **forestFloor** package (Welling et al. 2016). This package provides 3D graphics and also adds color gradients useful for investigating interactions between explanatory variables.

For the other monitoring stations, the code (omitted here, as well as the graphics) is very similar as before. Indeed, only the name of the station changes and data for the other stations are also available in the **VSURF** package. By examining the marginal effects of all variables on PM10 pollution for every monitoring station, the following conclusions can be drawn.

First of all, we can state a general remark: intensities of partial effects of meteorological variables are lower than those of pollutants. Indeed, consider a partial effect of one pollutant. Realizations of concentrations of the other pollutants integrate weather factors and lead to coherent evolutions between pollutants. This is why we will distinguish the effects of pollutants from those of the weather.

- *Effects of pollutants.* They are always increasing as expected, roughly linear in appearance, slightly convex or concave in shape depending on the pollutant and the station.
- *Rain effect.* It is always decreasing since it reflects a cleaning effect.

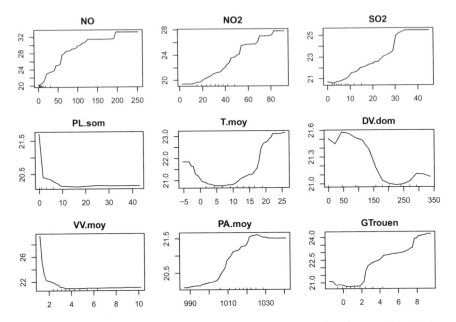

Fig. 3.13 Marginal effects of each variable on the PM10 concentration, from an RF trained on station JUS

- *Temperature effects.* These are nonlinear effects: positive when it is cold or hot, zero or negative when the temperature is average.
- *Effect of wind direction.* Two situations must be distinguished:
    - The one that is similar to JUS: GCM and AIL, where the effect of the wind direction shows an east/west axis.
    - Or as for GUI, REP, HRI, where the effect of the direction shows an inhibitory north/south axis.
- *Effect of wind speed.* It is necessary to distinguish three situations according to which the effect is inhibitory (for JUS and GUI) or decreasing (for GCM, REP, and HRI), what is expected, or even increasing for AIL. This is the only point that is, at first sight, surprising. It is explained by the absence of a local pollution source combined with a low level of pollution, which means that the main source is the import of pollution, hence the increasing effect of wind speed.
- *Effect of relative humidity.* Those effects are of very little importance and are very rarely useful in the rest of the work. The weak min and max effects are different: increasing and decreasing, respectively.
- *Effect of atmospheric pressure.* It is still growing as expected.
- *Effect of temperature gradient.* It is still growing as expected. The temperature gradients of Le Havre and Rouen give very similar and equally important information.

Conclusion

The main conclusion is twofold:

- The effects of pollutants are always increasing, and are therefore markers of local pollution useful for dust modeling.
- For weather variables, we distinguish (by eliminating HR which is of low importance)

  - Those that have a rather unfavorable (decreasing) effect on pollution: PL and VV (for all stations except AIL).
  - Those that have a favorable (increasing) effect: GT, PA, and VV (for AIL).
  - Those that have an unfavorable and then favorable effect: T (unfavorable if cold then favorable when it is not cold), DV.

This study on marginal effects will be supplemented by the relative importance of the variables (see Sect. 4.5.4).

Chapter 4
Variable Importance

Abstract Here, the focus is on creating a hierarchy of input variables, based on a quantification of the importance of their effects on the response variable. Such an index of importance provides a ranking of variables. Random forests offer an ideal framework, as they do not make any assumptions regarding the underlying model. This chapter introduces permutation variable importance using random forests and illustrates its use on the spam dataset. The behavior of the variable importance index is first studied with regard to data-related aspects: the number of observations, number of variables, and presence of groups of correlated variables. Then, its behavior with regard to random forest parameters is addressed. In the final section, the use of variable importance is first illustrated by simulation in regression, and then in three examples: predicting ozone concentration, analyzing genomic data, and determining the local level of dust pollution.

4.1 Notions of Importance

In this chapter, the focus is on constructing a hierarchy of explanatory variables based on a quantification of the importance of their effects on the response variable. Such an index of importance provides a ranking of variables, from the most important to the least important. A general discussion on variable importance can be found in Azen and Budescu (2003). This notion has been mainly studied in the context of linear models, as highlighted by Grömping (2015)'s review or Wallard (2015)'s PhD thesis. From this standpoint, random forests offer an ideal framework, as they are much more general and, as previously mentioned, do not make any assumptions regarding the underlying model. They combine a nonparametric method, which does not specify a particular type of the relationship between Y and X, with resampling to provide an efficient and convenient definition of such indices.

In this context, one of the most widely used measures of the importance of a given variable is the average (among trees in a forest) increase in the error made by

© Springer Nature Switzerland AG 2020
R. Genuer and J.-M. Poggi, *Random Forests with R*, Use R!,
https://doi.org/10.1007/978-3-030-56485-8_4

a tree when the observed values of that variable are randomly permuted in the OOB samples.

Definition 4.1 (*Variable importance*) Let us fix $j \in \{1, \ldots, p\}$ and calculate $VI(X^j)$, the importance index of variable X^j:

- Consider a bootstrap sample $\mathcal{L}_n^{\Theta_\ell}$ and the associated OOB_ℓ sample, that is, all observations that do not belong to $\mathcal{L}_n^{\Theta_\ell}$.
- Calculate errOOB$_\ell$, the error made on OOB_ℓ by the tree built on $\mathcal{L}_n^{\Theta_\ell}$ (mean square error or misclassification rate).
- Then randomly permute the values of variable X^j in the OOB_ℓ sample. This gives a perturbed sample, noted $\widetilde{OOB}_\ell^j$.
- Finally, calculate $\text{err}\widetilde{OOB}_\ell^j$, the error made on $\widetilde{OOB}_\ell^j$ by the tree built on $\mathcal{L}_n^{\Theta_\ell}$.
- Repeat these operations for all bootstrap samples. The importance of the variable X^j, $VI(X^j)$, is then defined by the difference between the average error of a tree on the perturbed OOB sample and that on the OOB sample:

$$
VI(X^j) = \frac{1}{q} \sum_{\ell=1}^{q} \left(\text{err}\widetilde{OOB}_\ell^j - \text{errOOB}_\ell \right).
$$

Thus, the higher the error increase originating from the random permutations of the variable, the more important is the variable. Conversely, if permutations have little or no effect on the error (or even cause a decrease, because VI can be slightly negative), the variable is considered unimportant.

This variable importance calculation above is exactly the one performed in the **randomForest** package. It should be noted that the definition of variable importance given by Breiman (2001) is slightly different. Indeed, if the perturbed OOB samples are obtained in the same way, the importance of a variable is defined by the difference between the OOB error on the perturbed OOB samples, and the initial OOB error. One possible explanation for this change could be the following. In the calculation of the OOB error, there is an aggregation step that tends to reduce individual trees' errors, so the use of the OOB error in the calculation tends to dampen the effects of random permutations of variables. However, when calculating importance, we want to magnify the effects of these permutations. Therefore, the OOB error is replaced by the average error on all trees, for which no aggregation step is performed.

Many studies, mainly by simulation, have been conducted to illustrate the behavior of RF variable importance, including (Strobl et al. 2007, 2008; Archer and Kimes 2008; Genuer et al. 2008, 2010b; Gregorutti et al. 2013). In this type of empirical work, it is often difficult to draw very confident general conclusions, but some interesting behaviors can be noted from this variable importance (VI henceforth) score that will be useful for variable selection:

- The VI variability, through repetitions, of variables outside the model is less than that of informative variables. Non-informative variables have a very low VI and their variation order of magnitude is useful for identifying them.

- In the presence of a group of highly correlated variables, masking effects appear but remain limited except when the number of variables in the group is dominant compared to other informative variables.
- A stable evaluation of these VI requires, on the one hand, large forests (with a high number of trees) and, on the other hand, some repetitions of such forests to be able to quantify their variability.

We will now focus on RF prediction performance by estimating the generalization error by out-of-bag error (OOB) and quantifying the permutation-based variable importance that are the main ingredients of our variable selection strategy, presented in Chap. 5.

To obtain the calculation of the permutation-based VI, it is necessary to add the option `importance = TRUE` in the `randomForest()` function:

```
> RFDefImp <- randomForest(type ~ ., data = spamApp,
    importance = TRUE)
> varImpPlot(RFDefImp, type = 1, scale = FALSE,
    n.var = ncol(spamApp) - 1, cex = 0.8,
    main = "Variable importance")
```

We can see in Fig. 4.1 a quantification of VI for `spam` data. It is both enlightening and easily interpretable. It makes it possible to identify very clearly a first group of variables: `capitalLong`, `remove`, `hp`, `charExclamation`, `capitalAve`, `capitalTotal`, `free`, and `charDollar` then, less clearly, a group of 8 variables which contains useful variables not only like `george` but also your or `number000` whose presence is less intuitive.

It may be noted that the most important variable (`capitalLong`) does not appear in any of the splits in the optimal tree, which proves that a variable that never comes out in the local minimization of heterogeneity can nevertheless be important because it is well correlated with all informative variables.

Remark 4.1 The `varImpPlot()` function of **randomForest** package allows to directly plot the importance of the variables classified in decreasing order of importance. However, we emphasize that we indicate `type = 1` because we only want to plot the permutation-based VI,[1] and `scale = FALSE` to get the raw importance, and not the normalized importance for which the average of the trees' errors is divided by the standard deviation of these errors.

In Gregorutti et al. (2015), the notion of permutation-based VI is directly extended to a group of variables. To do this, it suffices to permute, in the OOB samples involved in the VI definition (see Definition 4.1), not only one variable but jointly all the variables of the same group. For functional additive models, the theoretical results of Gregorutti et al. (2013) are extended. Then a strategy for selecting variables in a multivariate functional data framework is derived by selecting groups of variables

---

[1]The option `type = 2` allows obtaining the MDI importance, defined in the next paragraph.

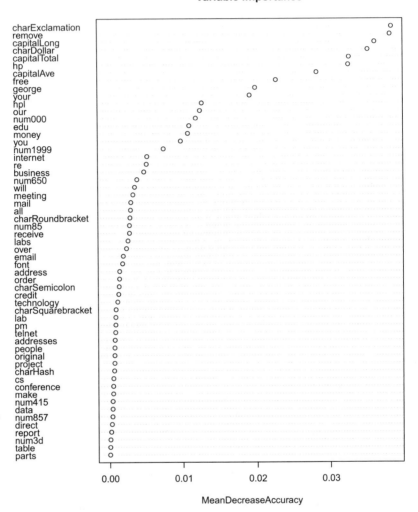

Fig. 4.1 Importance of variables ranked in descending order for spam data

made of wavelet coefficient sets, representing the different functional variables, and using a Recursive Feature Elimination (RFE) strategy. These tools are available in the **RFgroove** package (Gregorutti 2016).

Finally, the very recent work of Ramosaj and Pauly (2019) shows that, at least in the case where input variables are independent, the permutation-based VI is asymptotically unbiased.

MDI Importance
It should be noted that there is another VI index based on the Mean Decrease Impurity (MDI) and inspired by the variable importance defined in CART method (see Sect. 2.5.3). It is defined as follows (Breiman 2001): for a given variable, its MDI is the sum of the impurity decreases for all nodes where the variable is used to split, weighted by the proportion of individuals in the node, on average on all trees in the forest. Although its use seems less frequent, it has given rise to theoretical results (Louppe et al. 2013) and finds interesting practical applications despite real limitations. In particular, it is highly dependent on forest parameters, biased for non-pruned trees and finally the theoretical results only cover binary categorical variables.

4.2 Variable Importance Behavior

We illustrate the behavior of the permutation-based variable importance on a simulated dataset, called *toys*. Introduced by Weston et al. (2003), it is a binary classification problem ($Y \in \{-1, 1\}$), with 6 "true" variables (related to Y) and noise variables (independent of Y). For the latter, we will speak indifferently of variables that are out of model or not informative.

The 6 true variables are divided into two independent groups: variables V1, V2, and V3 on the one hand and variables V4, V5, and V6 on the other hand.

Definition 4.2 (*Toys* model) The simulation model is defined using the distribution of input variables X^j conditionally to $Y = y$ as follows:

- For 70% of the observations: $X^j \sim \mathcal{N}(y \times j, 1)$ for $j = 1, 2, 3$ and $X^j \sim \mathcal{N}(0, 1)$ for $j = 4, 5, 6$.
- For the remaining 30% of observations: $X^j \sim \mathcal{N}(0, 1)$ for $j = 1, 2, 3$ and $X^j \sim \mathcal{N}(y \times (j - 3), 1)$ for $j = 4, 5, 6$.

The additional noise variables, when $p > 6$, are generated independently of Y: $X^j \sim \mathcal{N}(0.1)$ for $j = 7, \ldots, p$.
Once simulated, the input variables are all standardized.

Figure 4.2 gives the histograms of the first 9 input variables for a simulation of 1,000 observations based on *toys* model. The definition of the *toys* model as well as the distribution of the input variables highlight the fact that the variables of the same group are sorted from the least related to Y to the most related to Y.

4.2.1 Behavior According to n and p

Starting from a classical situation with $n = 500$ and $p = 6$, illustrating a very good result of VI computation, we show in Fig. 4.3 the behavior of VI when increasing the number of input variables and also when decreasing the number of observations.

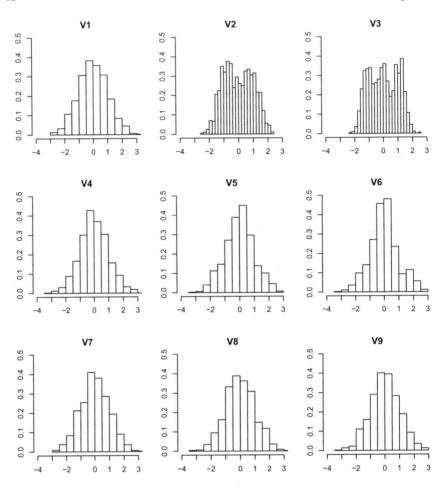

Fig. 4.2 Histograms of the first 9 input variables of *toys* model for a simulation of 1,000 observations

The graphs in the first row of Fig. 4.3 illustrate that in the case of a high number of observations, the importance of the variables behaves well (in the sense that V1 to V6 are the most important) even when the dimension increases. Indeed, even if the importance of the variables in the model decreases, they remain much higher than the importance of variables outside the model.

In the second row, we see that even in cases where $p > n$, the overall behavior remains satisfactory, even if importance of variable V4 no longer differs from out-of-model variables when $p = 200$ or $p = 500$. However, this variable is quite uninformative in this simulation model.

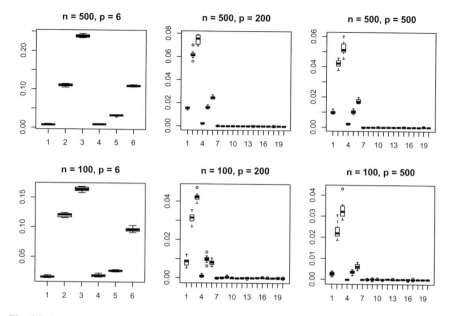

Fig. 4.3 Boxplots of the importance of variables (on 50 forests) according to n and p, *toys* model

4.2.2 Behavior for Groups of Correlated Variables

Let us take as a reference the case where $n = 100$ and $p = 200$, and simulate 1, 10, and then 20 variables linearly correlated with V3 (the most important variable of the first group {V1, V2, V3 }), with a correlation coefficient of 0.9. Importance scores of the first variables are represented in Fig. 4.4.

We notice that as the number of variables correlated with V3 increases, importance scores of the variables correlated with V3 (i.e., V1, V2, V3 and the "replicates" of V3) decreases. However, we see that even in cases where the size of the group of correlated variables is large (case with 20 variables), importance scores of V3 and of many variables in the group are still much larger than the ones of variables out of the model. Finally, we can also see that VI of variables V4, V5, V6 are not affected at all by additional variables correlated with V3.

Let us now consider the case where we simulate both variables linearly correlated with V3 and others with V6 (setting all correlation coefficients to 0.9). The results of this scenario are presented in Fig. 4.5.

In this case, we notice that the importance of the two groups of correlated variables decreases when variables, respectively, correlated with V3 and V6 are added. In addition, the relative importance of the two groups is quite respected and many variables in each of the two groups are still much important than variables outside the model.

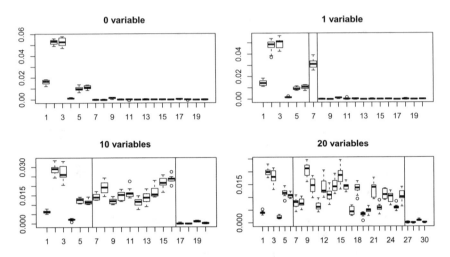

Fig. 4.4 Boxplots of the importance of the variables (on 50 forests) according to the number of variables correlated with V3, these being located between the two vertical lines, *toys* model

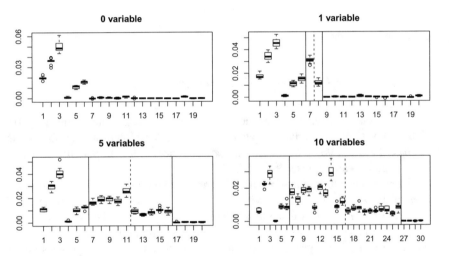

Fig. 4.5 Boxplots of the importance of the variables (over 50 forests) according to the size of the groups of variables correlated with V3 on the one hand and V6 on the other hand. The variables correlated with V3 are located between the left vertical line and the dotted vertical line, followed by those correlated with V6, *toys* model

4.3 Tree Diversity and Variables Importance

Let us go back to the simple case where we consider only stumps (two-leaf trees). In Sect. 3.5.2, we highlight the effect of `mtry` on the variables used in the root node.

Let us now focus on the effect of this tree diversity on variable importance, by again building a Bagging predictor only made of stumps on `spam` data, but now with VI computation:

```
> bagStumpImp <- randomForest(type ~ ., spamApp,
    mtry = ncol(spamApp) - 1, maxnodes = 2, importance = TRUE)
> varImpPlot(bagStumpImp, type = 1, scale = FALSE, n.var = 20,
    cex = 0.8, main = "Variable importance")
```

In Fig. 4.6, we observe that almost all the variables are of no importance, and we only detect variables `charExclamation` and `charDollar`, which is consistent with the fact that only these two variables are actually used to split the root node.

Now let us compare it to an RF only made of stumps, built with the default value of `mtry` (equal to 7 here):

```
> RFStumpImp <- randomForest(type ~ ., spamApp, maxnodes = 2,
    importance = TRUE)
> varImpPlot(RFStumpImp, type = 1, scale = FALSE, n.var = 20,
    cex = 0.8, main = "Variable importance")
```

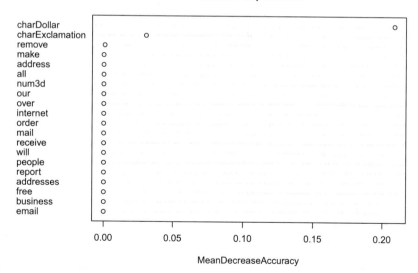

Fig. 4.6 Importance of the 20 most important variables for a Bagging of stumps, `spam` data

Variable importance

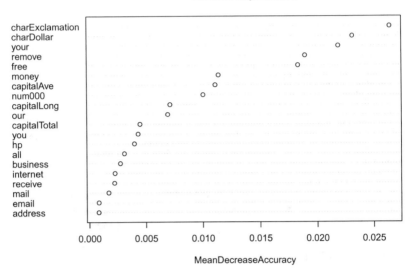

Fig. 4.7 Importance of the 20 most important variables for an RF of stumps with the default value of `mtry` (equal to 7), `spam` data

We observe (Fig. 4.7) that many more variables are of strictly positive importance (the randomization at the variable level actually changes the subset of variables chosen at each node to participate in the split). Moreover, the variables that emerge with the greatest importance are almost the same as those from an RF with maximal trees, ignoring the order. Thus, even with trees that are clearly not complex enough, RF can retrieve the interesting information contained in the variables.

4.4 Influence of Parameters on Variable Importance

If the only goal is to achieve good predictive performance with RF, we recommend adjusting the RF parameters based on the OOB error. However, when we also wish to have information on the variables, or even to select variables, we must try to adjust the RF parameters by looking at their impact on VI.

We illustrate the behavior of VI as a function of parameters in the *toys* simulation model. We start from the framework where $n = 100$ and $p = 200$ and represent in Fig. 4.8 the VI obtained by varying the number of trees `ntree` (on rows) and the `mtry` parameter (on columns).

Increasing the number of trees has the effect of stabilizing the VI, and the default value 500 seems large enough in this example. On the other hand, when the value of `mtry` increases, we notice that the importance of the most influential variables of the model increases, with a very large increase when going from 14 (which is

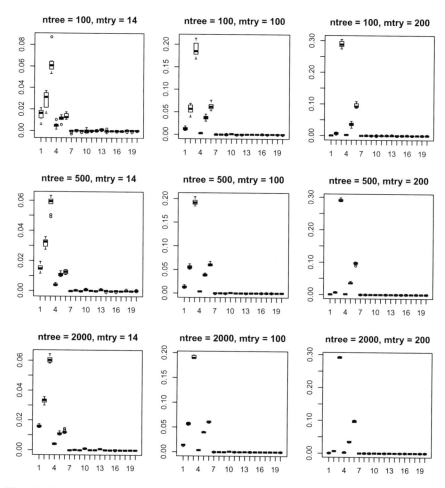

Fig. 4.8 Boxplot of the importance of the variables (on 50 forests) according to `ntree` and `mtry`, *toys* model

the default value of `randomForest()`) to 100. Finally, we also see a stabilization effect of VI when the value of `mtry` increases.

Thus, in a very parsimonious case such as the one studied here (6 variables related to Y among 200), it seems necessary to increase the value of `mtry` in order to stabilize importance of model variables and to help highlighting the most influential variables.

4.5 Examples

4.5.1 An Illustration by Simulation in Regression

We use a simple example in regression, to illustrate the use of variable importance in this context, as well as the use of partial effects (defined in Sect. 3.6.3). In this classic example introduced in Friedman (1991) and accessible *via* the **mlbench** package, observations are generated by the following model:

$$Y = 10 \sin(\pi \, X1 \, X2) + 20(X3 - 0.5)^2 + 10 \, X4 + 5 \, X5 + \varepsilon$$

and in which there are 10 input variables assumed independent and with the same uniform distribution on [0, 1]. Thus, only 5 of them are actually used to generate the outputs and, moreover, it is assumed that $\varepsilon \sim \mathcal{N}(0, 1)$.

Let us simulate 500 observations using the model and build an RF with VI computation:

```
> library(mlbench)
> fried1Simu <- mlbench.friedman1(n = 500)
> fried1Data <- data.frame(fried1Simu$x, y = fried1Simu$y)
> fried1RFimp <- randomForest(y ~ ., fried1Data, importance = TRUE)
> varImpPlot(fried1RFimp, type = 1, scale = FALSE,
     main = "Variable importance")
```

Variable importance (Fig. 4.9) clearly identifies the 5 variables in the model that actually contribute to response computation and discards the non-informative variables.

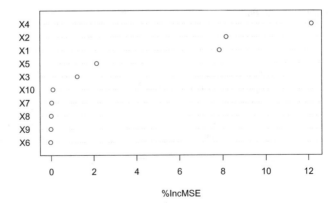

Fig. 4.9 Importance of variables, simulated data in regression

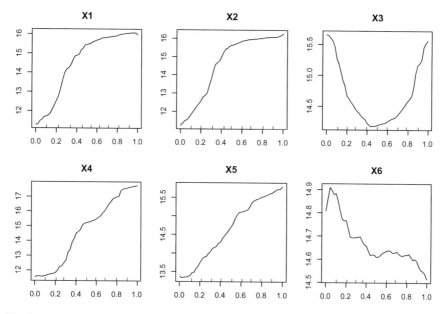

Fig. 4.10 Marginal effects, simulated data in regression

Recall that to obtain the partial effect, for example, of variable $X1$, we use the following command:

```
> partialPlot(fried1RFimp, fried1Data, x.var = "X1", main = "X1")
```

Partial effects of the first 6 variables (Fig. 4.10) allow finding a very weak effect of the sixth, almost perfectly linear effects for $X4$ and $X5$, a quadratic effect for $X3$ and identical effects for $X1$ and $X2$ which are the best additive approximation of the first term of the regression function $10\sin(\pi\ X1\ X2)$.

4.5.2 *Predicting Ozone Concentration*

For a presentation of this dataset, see Sect. 1.5.2.

Let us load the **randomForest** package and `Ozone` data, then build an RF with the default parameters and permutation-based VI computation:

```
> library("randomForest")
> data("Ozone", package = "mlbench")
> OzRFDefImp <- randomForest(V4 ~ ., Ozone, na.action = na.omit,
    importance = TRUE)
```

The plot of VI obtained using the `varImpPlot()` function is given in Fig. 4.11:

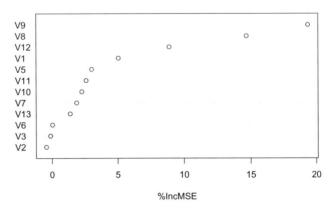

Fig. 4.11 Importance of variables, obtained with a default RF, Ozone data

```
> varImpPlot(OzRFDefImp, type = 1, scale = FALSE,
    main = "Variable importance")
```

This dataset has already been the subject of many studies and, even if they are real data, it is possible to know a priori which variables are supposed to be the most important and, on the other hand, which are the main sources of nonlinearity.

As noted in previous studies, three groups of very easily interpretable variables can be identified, ranging from the most important to the least important:

- The first group contains the two temperatures (V8 and V9) and the inversion base temperature (V12), known to be the best ozone predictors, and the month number (V1), which is an important predictor since ozone concentration has a strong seasonal component.
- The second group of significantly less important meteorological variables includes pressure height (V5), humidity (V7), basic inversion height (V10), pressure gradient (V11), and visibility (V13).
- Finally, the last group contains three irrelevant variables: the day of the month (V2), the day of the week (V3) as expected, and more surprisingly the wind speed (V6). The latter is a classic fact: the wind only enters the model when ozone pollution occurs, otherwise wind and pollution are weakly correlated and since most of the time pollution levels are moderate, this explains the low overall importance of the wind.

Let us go back to V2 which appeared high in the default tree obtained in Fig. 2.10. Variable importance thus shows a very satisfactory behavior by eliminating the effects of the selection bias of this variable in the splits.

Finally, as we noticed in Sect. 3.6.1, in this example, the OOB error increases with mtry, which is unusual. This can be explained by studying the behavior of the

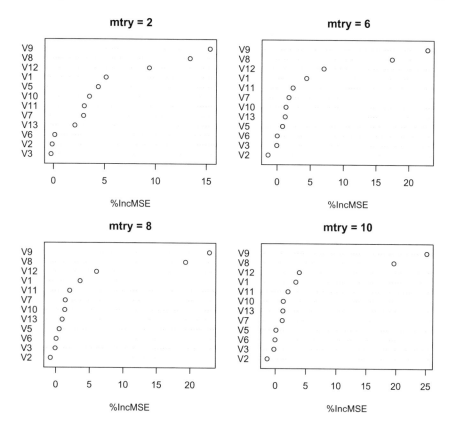

Fig. 4.12 Evolution of VI as a function of mtry, `Ozone` data

importance of variables as a function of `mtry`. Figure 4.12 contains the VI plots for `mtry` values of {2, 6, 8, 10}, while Fig. 4.11 contains the one for `mtry` = 4.

Note that as soon as `mtry` equals 4, the probability that one of the variables among {`V9`, `V8`, `V12`, `V10`} belongs to the randomly selected variables set in a node (before the best split is determined) is increasingly high. These four variables being highly correlated with each other and also highly correlated with the response variable `V4` (Table 4.1) results is a very low tree diversity as soon as `mtry` equals 4, and which decreases further as `mtry` increases.

4.5.3 Analyzing Genomic Data

For a presentation of this dataset, see Sect. 1.5.3.

Let us load the **randomForest** package and `vac18` data:

Table 4.1 Variable correlation matrix V4, V8, V9, V10, and V12, Ozone data

	V4	V8	V9	V10	V12
V4	1.00	0.76	0.75	−0.54	0.70
V8	0.76	1.00	0.91	−0.51	0.84
V9	0.75	0.91	1.00	−0.59	0.93
V10	−0.54	−0.51	−0.59	1.00	−0.79
V12	0.70	0.84	0.93	−0.79	1.00

```
> library(randomForest)
> data("vac18", package = "mixOmics")
```

Then let us create an object `geneExpr` containing the gene expressions and an object `stimu` containing the stimuli to be predicted:

```
> geneExpr <- vac18$genes
> stimu <- vac18$stimulation
```

An RF, computing permutation-based VI and with the `mtry` parameter set to $p/3$ (as mentioned in Sect. 3.6.2, the default value, equal to 31, is too low for this high-dimensional dataset) is obtained as follows:

```
> vacRFDefImp <- randomForest(x = geneExpr, y = stimu,
      mtry = ncol(geneExpr)/3, importance = TRUE)
```

The `varImpPlot()` function returns by default the importance of the variables for the 30 most important variables (see Fig. 4.13):

```
> varImpPlot(vacRFDefImp, type = 1, scale = FALSE, cex = 0.8)
```

A plot of VI of all variables (representation used in Chap. 5) can be obtained with the following commands:

```
> vacImp <- vacRFDefImp$importance[, nlevels(stimu) + 1]
> plot(sort(vacImp, decreasing = TRUE), type = "l",
      xlab = "Variables", ylab = "Variable importance")
```

The shape of the curve plotted in Fig. 4.14 is quite standard in high dimension and highlights a very strong sparsity for `Vac18` data. Indeed, we see that only a small number of variables have a significantly positive VI score.

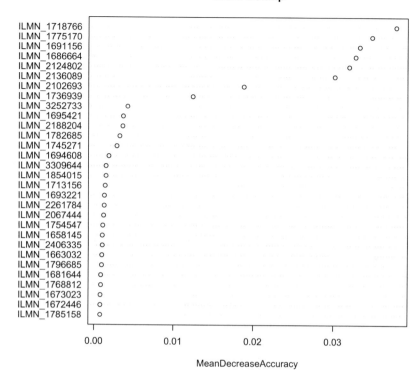

Fig. 4.13 Importance of the 30 most important variables sorted in descending order, `Vac18` data

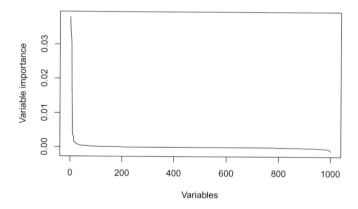

Fig. 4.14 Importance of all variables sorted in descending order of importance, `Vac18` data

4.5.4   Air Pollution by Dust: What Is the Local Contribution?

We continue here the example of dust pollution in the network of the Haute-Normandie region (Sect. 3.6.3), this time taking inspiration from the work of Bobbia et al. (2011). We do not provide details on the R code used in this part, but prefer to show another example of the possible use of variable importance.

In France, several regional plans have been defined to reduce pollution. In this context, determining the local contribution in relation to the background contribution of a specific pollution is necessary. This makes it possible to assess the proportion of pollution on which it is possible to act and can help to adapt the regional plan. An assessment of the local contribution can be carried out using deterministic models that provide a pollution map of the entire country at a regional scale. They are not related to pollution measurements at monitoring sites but depend on imprecise and difficult to obtain emissions inventory. The large uncertainties that result from this therefore lead to the use of statistical tools rather than a purely deterministic approach. An example of such an approach has recently been conducted in the Haute-Normandie region to quantify local and background contributions specifically to dust pollution.

In the first step, the marginal effects were classified according to the characteristics of the monitoring stations: some are close to traffic, others measure urban or industrial background pollution, and the last is located in a rural area. Local pollution is thus characterized by conventional pollutants, including nitrogen oxides for urban pollution and sulfur dioxide for industrial use. It should be recalled that three groups of meteorological variables have been structured in the following way-those with an adverse effect on pollution: PL and VV (for all stations except AIL); a positive effect: GT, PA, and VV (for AIL); and a non-monotonic effect: T, DV.

Then, for each of the six monitoring stations, the individual VI is computed using an RF model containing a large number of variables. To define the importance of a group of variables, we propose to adopt the following rule: if the variables of the group are redundant (either well correlated or, more weakly, with similar "effects on PM10 concentrations") then the importance of the group is defined by the maximum individual VI in this group. In this way, groups of variables can be directly compared. The results are summarized in Table 4.2.

The importance of the three groups of weather variables is almost equal to 20, with the exception of PA for GUI which reaches 32. On the other hand, the importance of pollutants (by restricting ourselves to the largest importance) fluctuates much more: from 28 to 49 if we exclude AIL since no measurement of pollutants were made there.

The two traffic stations (GUI and REP) give close values for the NO2 importance (41 and 45). The two urban stations (JUS and HRI), on the other hand, have different importance for SO2: 28 and 49, respectively. For the industrial station (GCM), the importance of the pollutant (SO2) is 39, which is intermediate.

The idea is to use the pollution from the AIL station (noted as PM10_AIL) as a measure of diffuse pollution at the regional level. It is supposed to capture phenomena on a more or less large scale (regional or more) and not be affected by significant

Table 4.2 Importance of variables, through stations, for pollutants and meteorological variables by group, where def means that the effect is unfavorable (increasing), fav that it is favorable (decreasing), and def-fav for non-monotonic effects on PM10 pollution

	Pollutants	Meteo def	Meteo fav	Meteo def-fav
GCM Rouen	39 (SO2)	23 (PL)	20 (GT)	21 (T)
JUS Rouen	28 (NO2)	19 (PL)	21 (GT)	19 (DV)
	22 (SO2)			
GUI Rouen	41 (NO2)	18 (PL)	32 (PA)	19 (T)
	18 (SO2)			
AIL Dieppe		15 (PL)	23 (PA)	21 (DV)
REP Le Havre	45 (NO2)	20 (VV)	24 (GT)	19 (T)
	31 (SO2)			
HRI Le Havre	22 (NO2)	16 (VV)	18 (GT)	22 (T)
	49 (SO2)			

Table 4.3 Importance scores of variables, through stations, for pollutants and meteorological variables by group, by adding PM10_AIL in the RF model

	Pollutants	Meteo def	Meteo fav	Meteo def-fav	PM10_AIL
GCM	33 (SO2)	23 (PL)	17 (GT)	16 (DV)	68
JUS	31 (NO)	19 (PL)	16 (GT)	13 (DV)	78
	18 (SO2)				
GUI	40 (NO2)	18 (PL)	26 (PA)	20 (T)	64
	17 (SO2)				
REP	28 (SO2)	18 (VV)	19 (GT)	12 (T)	81
	44 (NO2)				
HRI	41 (SO2)	12 (VV)	11 (GT)	13 (T)	86
	14 (NO)				

local production. This is supported by examining the concentration distributions at all stations for days when PM10_AIL exceeds 30 (33 days are concerned): the median is around 40 and the first quartile around 33.

The computation of the importance of variable PM10_AIL in previous models when completed by the introduction of this new variable leads to the results recorded in Table 4.3:

- Its importance is in the order of 64 to 86, which is considerable.
- The importance of pollutants fluctuates a little bit, and this is for all stations.
- The importance of weather variables decreases significantly.

These elements are consistent with the idea that PM10 concentrations at AIL reflect diffuse pollution in the sense that it does not perturb the importance of local markers while it affects the importance of weather variables.

Table 4.4 Importance of variables, through stations, for pollutants and after replacing meteorological variables by PM10_AIL in forest variables

	Main pollutant	Other pollutants	PM10_AIL
GCM	73 (SO2)		98
JUS	35 (NO)	26, 22 (NO2, SO2)	89
GUI	42 (NO2)	31, 20 (NO, SO2)	77
REP	42 (SO2)	41, 36 (NO2, NO)	78
HRI	50 (SO2)	21, 19 (NO, NO2)	81

For each of the other five stations, an RF is then trained with VI computation based on available pollutants and PM10 concentrations at AIL only. This eliminates all weather variables. The results of the importance are gathered in Table 4.4.

All partial effects are generally increasing and weakly nonlinear (except sometimes for extreme SO2 levels). The interpretation is as follows: by introducing this variable, which seems to capture a kind of diffuse pollution by dust, the model is almost linearized.

In conclusion, thanks to such a method, it has been possible to consider that in the Haute-Normandie region, the importance of the local share of dust pollution, which can be controlled by regulatory measures, does not generally exceed that of large-scale pollution.

Chapter 5
Variable Selection

Abstract This chapter is dedicated to variable selection using random forests: an automatic three-step procedure involving first a fairly coarse elimination of a large number of useless variables, followed by a finer and ascending sequential introduction of variables into random forest models, for interpretation and then for prediction. The principle and the procedure implemented in the VSURF package are presented on the spam dataset. The choice of VSURF parameters suitable for selection is then studied. In the final section, the variable selection procedure is applied to two real examples: predicting ozone concentration and analyzing genomic data.

5.1 Generalities

In the past, classic statistical problems typically involved many observations ($n =$, e.g., a few hundred or a few thousand) and relatively a few variables ($p =$ one to a few tens). Today, the ease of data acquisition has led to huge databases that collect new information almost daily. Traditional statistical techniques are poorly suited to processing these new quantities of data, in which the number of variables p can reach tens or even hundreds of thousands. At the same time, for many applications, the number of observations n can be reduced to a few tens, e.g., in the case of biomedical data. In this context, it is indeed common to gather many types of data on a given individual (e.g., gene expression data), but to keep the number of individuals on whom the experiment is conducted small (for the study of a disease, the number of affected individuals included in the study is often very limited). These data are said to be of high dimension: the number of variables is quite large in comparison to the number of observations, which is classically denoted by $n \ll p$. Here, we are referring to problems where n is several hundreds and p is several thousands. One of the most attractive features of random forests is that they are highly efficient both for traditional problems (where $p \leq n$) and for such high-dimensional problems. Indeed, RF have been previously shown to be inherently adapted to the high-dimensional case. For instance, Biau (2012) shows that if the true model meets certain sparsity conditions, then the RF predictor depends only on the active variables.

© Springer Nature Switzerland AG 2020
R. Genuer and J.-M. Poggi, *Random Forests with R*, Use R!,
https://doi.org/10.1007/978-3-030-56485-8_5

In many situations, in addition to designing a good predictor, practitioners also want additional information on the variables used in the problem. Statisticians are invited to propose a selection of variables in order to identify those that are most useful in explaining the input–output relationship. In this context, it is natural to think that relatively a few variables (say at most n and hopefully much less, for example, $\sqrt{n}$) actually affect the output, and it is necessary to make additional assumptions (called parsimony or sparsity) to make it tractable and meaningful. In Giraud (2014), there is a very complete presentation of mathematical problems and techniques for addressing this kind of questions.

Let us mention some methods for variable selection in high-dimensional contexts. Starting with an empirical study in Poggi and Tuleau (2006) where a method based on the variable importance index provided by the CART algorithm is introduced. In the same flavor, let us also mention Questier et al. (2005). Considering the problem more generally, Guyon et al. (2002), Rakotomamonjy (2003), and Ghattas and Ben Ishak (2008) use the score provided by the Support Vector Machines (SVM: Vapnik 2013) and Díaz-Uriarte and Alvarez De Andres (2006) propose a variable selection procedure based on the variable importance index related to random forests. These methods calculate a score for each of the variables, then perform a sequential introduction of variables (*forward* methods), or a sequential elimination of variables (*backward* or RFE for Recursive Feature Elimination methods), or perform step-by-step methods (*stepwise* methods) combining introduction and elimination of variables. In Fan and Lv (2008), a two-step method is proposed: a first step of eliminating variables to reach a reasonable situation where p is of the same order of magnitude of n, then a second step of model building using a forward strategy based, for example, on the Least Absolute Shrinkage and Selection Operator (Lasso: Tibshirani 1996). In this spirit, a general scheme for calculating an importance score for variables is proposed in Lê Cao et al. (2007), then the authors use this scheme with CART and SVM as the base method. Their idea is to learn a weight vector on all variables (their meta-algorithm is called Optimal Feature Weighting, OFW): a variable with a large weight is important, while a variable with a small weight is useless.

Finally, more recently, methods to improve Lasso for variable selection have been developed. The latter have points in common with the ensemble methods. Indeed, instead of trying to make selection "at once" with a classic Lasso, the idea is to construct several subsets of variables and then combine them. In Bolasso (for Bootstrap-enhanced Lasso), introduced by Bach (2008), several bootstrap samples are generated and then the Lasso method is applied to each of them. Bolasso is therefore to be compared with the Bagging of Breiman (1996). In Randomized Lasso, Meinshausen and Bühlmann (2010) propose to generate several samples by subsampling and add an additional random perturbation to the construction of the Lasso itself. Randomized Lasso is therefore to be compared to Random Forests-RI variant of random forests. In the same spirit, we can also mention Fellinghauer et al. (2013) which use RF for robust estimation in graphical models.

Interest in the subject still continues: for example, Hapfelmeier and Ulm (2012) propose a new selection approach using RF, and Cadenas et al. (2013) describe and compare these different approaches in a survey paper.

5.2 Principle

In Genuer et al. (2010b), we propose a variable selection method (see also in Genuer et al. 2015, the corresponding **VSURF** package). This is an automatic procedure in the sense that there is no a priori to make the selection. For example, it is not necessary to specify the desired number of variables; the procedure adapts to the data to provide the final subset of variables. The method involves two steps: the first, fairly coarse and descending, proceeds by thresholding the importance of the variables to eliminate a large number of useless variables, while the second, finer and ascending, consists of a sequential introduction of variables into random forest models.

In addition, we distinguish two variable selection objectives: interpretation and prediction (although this terminology may lead to confusion):

- For interpretation, we try to select all the variables X^j strongly related to the response variable Y (even if the variables X^j are correlated with each other).
- While for a prediction purpose, we try to select a parsimonious subset of variables sufficient to properly predict the response variable.

Typically, a subset built to satisfy the first objective may contain many variables, which will potentially be highly correlated with each other. On the contrary, a subset of variables satisfying the second one will contain a few variables, weakly correlated.

A situation illustrates the distinction between the two types of variable selection. Consider a high-dimensional classification problem ($n \ll p$) for which each explanatory variable is associated with a pixel in an image or a voxel in a 3D image as in brain activity classification (fMRI) problems; see, for example Genuer et al. (2010a). In such situations, it is natural to assume that many variables are useless or uninformative and that there are unknown groups of highly correlated predictors corresponding to regions of the brain involved in the response to a given stimulation. Although both variable selection objectives may be of interest in this case, it is clear that finding all the important variables highly related to the response variable is useful for interpretation, since the selected variables correspond to entire regions of the brain or of an image. Of course, the search for a small number of variables, sufficient for a good prediction, makes it possible to obtain the most discriminating variables in the regions previously highlighted but is of less priority in this context.

5.3 Procedure

In this section, we present the skeleton of the procedure before providing additional details, in the next section, after the application of the method to the `spam` data.

The first step is common to both objectives while the second depends on the goal:

- Step 1. Ranking and preliminary elimination:

  - Rank the variables by decreasing importance (in fact by average VI over typically 50 forests).
  - Eliminate the variables of low importance (let us denote m to be the number of retained variables).

    More precisely, starting from this order, we consider the corresponding sequence of standard deviations of the VIs that we use to estimate a threshold value on the VIs. Since the variability of the VIs is greater for the variables truly in the model than for the uninformative variables, the threshold value is given by estimating the standard deviation of the VI for the latter variables. This threshold is set at the minimum predicted value given by the CART model fitting the data (X, Y) where the Y are the standard deviations of the VI and the X are their ranks.

    Then only variables whose average importance VI is greater than this threshold are kept.

- Step 2. Variable selection:

  - For *interpretation*: we build the collection of nested models given by forests built on the data restricted to the first k variables (that is the k most important), for $k = 1$ to m, and we select the variables of the model leading to the lowest OOB error. Let us denote by m' the number of selected variables.

    More precisely, we calculate the averages (typically over 25 forests) of the OOB errors of the nested models starting with the one with only the most important variable and ending with the one involving all the important variables previously selected. Ideally, the variables of the model leading to the lowest OOB error are selected. In fact, to deal with instability, we use a classical trick: we select the smallest model with an error less than the lowest OOB error plus an estimate of the standard deviation of this error (based on the same 25 RF).

  - For *prediction*: from the variables selected for interpretation, a sequence of models is constructed by sequentially introducing the variables in increasing order of importance and iteratively testing them. The variables of the last model are finally selected.

    More precisely, the sequential introduction of variables is based on the following test: a variable is added only if the OOB error decreases more than a threshold. The idea is that the OOB error must decrease more than the average variation generated by the inclusion of non-informative variables. The threshold is set to the average of the absolute values of the first-order differences of the OOB errors between the models including m' variables and the one with m variables:

$$\frac{1}{m - m'} \sum_{j=m'}^{m-1} | err\,OOB(j+1) - err\,OOB(j) | \qquad (5.1)$$

where $err\,OOB(j)$ is the OOB error of the forest built with the j most important variables.

It should be stressed that all thresholds and reference values are calculated using only the data and do not have to be set in advance.

5.4 The VSURF Package

Let us start by illustrating the use of the **VSURF** package (Variable Selection Using Random Forests) on the simulated data *toys* introduced in Sect. 4.2 with $n = 100$ and $p = 200$, i.e., 6 true variables and 194 non-informative variables. The loading of the **VSURF** package as well as the `toys` data, included in the package, is done using the following commands:

```
> library(VSURF)
> data("toys")
```

The VSURF() function is the main function of the package and performs all the steps of the procedure. The random seed is fixed in order to obtain exactly the same results when applying later the procedure step by step:

```
> set.seed(3101318)
> vsurfToys <- VSURF(toys$x, toys$y, mtry = 100)
```

The methods `print()`, `summary()`, and `plot()` provide information on the results:

```
> summary(vsurfToys)

  VSURF computation time: 1.2 mins

  VSURF selected:
     34 variables at thresholding step (in 45 secs)
     4 variables at interpretation step (in 24.7 secs)
     3 variables at prediction step (in 1.2 secs)
```

```
> plot(vsurfToys)
```

Now, let us detail the main steps of the procedure using the results obtained on simulated `toys` data. Unless explicitly stated otherwise, all graphs refer to Fig. 5.1.

- Step 1.

  - Variable ranking.
    The result of the ranking of the variables is drawn on the graph at the top left. Informative variables are significantly more important than noise variables.
  - Variable elimination.
    From this ranking, we construct the curve of the corresponding standard deviations of VIs. This curve is used to estimate a threshold value for VIs. This

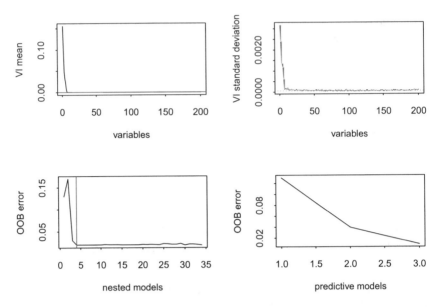

Fig. 5.1 Illustration of the results of the VSURF() function applied to the toys data

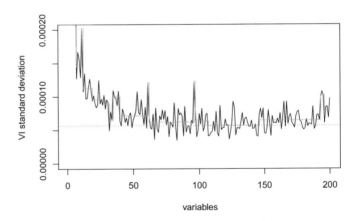

Fig. 5.2 Zoom of the top-right graph of Fig. 5.1

threshold (represented by the horizontal dotted red line in Fig. 5.2, which is a
zoom of the top-right graph of Fig. 5.1), is set to the minimum predicted value
given by a CART model fitted to this curve (see the piecewise constant green
function on the same graph).

We then retain only the variables whose average VI exceeds this threshold, i.e.,
those whose VI is above the horizontal red line in the graph at the top left of
Fig. 5.1.

The construction of forests and the ranking and elimination steps are obtained using the VSURF_thres() function:

```
> set.seed(3101318)
> vsurfThresToys <- VSURF_thres(toys$x, toys$y, mtry = 100)
```

The output of the VSURF_thres() function is a list containing all the results of this step. The main output arguments are varselect.thres which contains the indices of the variables selected at this step, imp.mean.dec and imp.sd.dec which contain the mean VI and the associated standard deviation (the order induced by the decreasing values of the mean VI is available in imp.mean.dec.ind).

```
> vsurfThresToys$varselect.thres
```

```
 [1]    3    2    6    5    1    4  184   37  138   81  159   17  180
[14]  191  131   94   52  165   96  192  157  198   21  111   25   29
[27]   12  109   64  107   70  186   46  188
```

Finally, Fig. 5.2 can be obtained directly from the object vsurfToys with the following command:

```
> plot(vsurfToys, step = "thres", imp.mean = FALSE,
       ylim = c(0, 2e-04))
```

We can see on the VI standard deviation curve (top-right graph of Fig. 5.1) that the standard deviation of the informative variables is large compared to that of the noise variables, which is close to zero.

- Step 2.

  – Procedure for selecting variables for interpretation.
    We calculate the OOB errors of random forests (on average over 25 repetitions) of nested models from the one with only the most important variable, and ending with the one with all the important variables stored previously.
    We select the smallest model with an OOB error less than the minimum OOB error increased by its empirical standard deviation (based on 25 repetitions).
    We use the VSURF_interp() function for this step. Note that we must specify the indices of the variables selected in the previous step, so we set the argument vars to vsurfThresToys$varselect.thres:

```
> vsurfInterpToys <- VSURF_interp(toys$x, toys$y,
      vars = vsurfThresToys$varselect.thres)
```

The list of results of the VSURF_interp() function gives access mainly to varselect.interp giving the variables selected by this step and err.interp containing the OOB errors of the nested RF models.

```
> vsurfInterpToys$varselect.interp
```

```
[1] 3 2 6 5
```

In the bottom-left graph, we see that the error is decreasing rapidly. It reaches almost its minimum when the first four true variables are included in the model (see the red vertical line), then it remains almost constant. The selected model contains the variables V3, V2, V6, and V5, which are four of the six true variables, while the real minimum is reached for 35 variables.

Note that, to ensure the quality of OOB error estimates (see Genuer et al. 2008) along nested RF models, the `mtry` parameter of the `randomForest()` function is set to its default value if k (the number of variables involved in the current RF model) is not greater than n, otherwise it is set to $k/3$.

– Variable selection procedure for prediction.

We perform a sequential introduction of variables with a test: a variable is added only if the accuracy gain exceeds a certain threshold. This is set so that the error reduction is significantly greater than the average variation obtained by adding noise variables.

We use the `VSURF_pred()` function for this step. We must specify the error rates and variables selected in the interpretation step, respectively, in `err.interp` and `varselect.interp` arguments:

```
> vsurfPredToys <- VSURF_pred(toys$x, toys$y,
      err.interp = vsurfInterpToys$err.interp,
      varselect.interp = vsurfInterpToys$varselect.interp)
```

The main outputs of the `VSURF_pred()` function are the variables selected by this last step, `varselect.pred`, and the OOB error rates of the RF models, `err.pred`.

```
> vsurfPredToys$varselect.pred
```

```
[1] 3 6 5
```

For `toys` data, the final model for prediction purposes only includes variables V3, V6, and V5 (see the graph at the bottom right). The threshold is set to the average of the absolute values of the differences of OOB error between the model with the $m' = 4$ variables and the model with $m = 36$ variables.

Finally, it should be noted that `VSURF_thres()` and `VSURF_interp()` can be executed in parallel using the same syntax as `VSURF()` (by specifying `parallel = TRUE`), while the `VSURF_pred()` function is not parallelizable.

Let us end this section by applying `VSURF()` to `spam` data.

Even if it is a dataset of moderate size, the strategy proposed here is quite time-consuming, so we will use `VSURF()` by taking advantage of parallel capabilities:

```
> set.seed(923321, kind = "L'Ecuyer-CMRG")
> vsurfSpam <- VSURF(type ~ ., spamApp, parallel = TRUE,
    ncores = 3, clusterType = "FORK")
```

The option `parallel = TRUE` allows to run the procedure in parallel, and the argument `clusterType` sets the type of "cluster" used: it can be left by default most of the time but the option `"FORK"` (specific to Linux and MacOS systems), coupled with the option `kind = "L'Ecuyer-CMRG"` of the `set.seed()` function , allows reproducibility of results.

```
> summary(vsurfSpam)

  VSURF computation time: 42.1 mins

  VSURF selected:
     55 variables at thresholding step (in 12.7 mins)
     24 variables at interpretation step (in 20.6 mins)
     19 variables at prediction step (in 8.7 mins)

  VSURF ran in parallel on a FORK cluster and used 3 cores
```

The overall calculation time is 42 min and the interpretation phase is the longest (half that of the total duration) while the other phases share the other half. The procedure identifies three sets of variables of decreasing size: 55, 24, and 19 and the results are summarized in Fig. 5.3.

```
> plot(vsurfSpam)
```

Let us focus on the 24 variables retained in the interpretation set. They are not surprising, at least for the first ones, but they are still numerous.

```
> colnames(spamApp[vsurfSpam$varselect.interp])
 [1] "remove"          "hp"              "capitalLong"
 [4] "charExclamation" "capitalAve"      "charDollar"
 [7] "capitalTotal"    "free"            "george"
[10] "num000"          "edu"             "your"
[13] "hpl"             "money"           "you"
[16] "our"             "business"        "num1999"
[19] "meeting"         "re"              "font"
[22] "num650"          "internet"        "receive"
```

If we move on to the 19 variables selected for prediction, there are hardly any fewer, but the ones that are eliminated, `num000`, `hpl`, `money`, `internet` and `receive`, are either weakly interesting (the last ones) or highly correlated with those retained (the other ones).

```
> colnames(spamApp[vsurfSpam$varselect.pred])
```

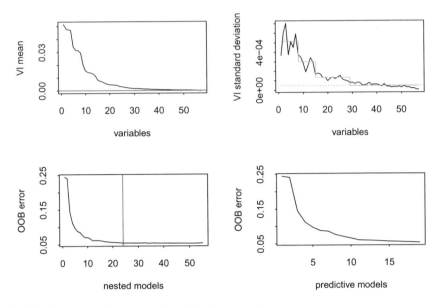

Fig. 5.3 Illustration of the results of VSURF(), spam data

```
[1]  "remove"           "hp"             "capitalLong"
[4]  "charExclamation"  "capitalAve"     "charDollar"
[7]  "capitalTotal"     "free"           "george"
[10] "edu"              "your"           "you"
[13] "our"              "business"       "num1999"
[16] "meeting"          "re"             "font"
[19] "num650"
```

Nevertheless, it is clear that our procedure keeps too many variables and this is related to the too small value of the average jump for the example spam:

```
> vsurfSpam$mean.jump
```
```
[1] 0.0002715288
```

Multiplying this value by 15 (fixed after a trial and error process) gives a more satisfactory result with 8 variables sufficient for the prediction which are all significant except the last one our.

```
> set.seed(945834)
> vsurfSpamPred <- VSURF_pred(type ~ ., spamApp, nmj = 15,
    err.interp = vsurfSpam$err.interp,
    varselect.interp = vsurfSpam$varselect.interp)
```

```
> colnames(spamApp[vsurfSpamPred$varselect.pred])
```
```
[1] "remove"      "capitalLong"   "charExclamation" "capitalAve"
[5] "charDollar"  "free"          "george"          "our"
```

5.5 Parameter Setting for Selection

First of all, since VSURF() is strongly based on randomForest(), the two main
parameters of this function (mtry and ntree) are taken over and have been kept
the same name, so everything that applies to RF also applies to VSURF() for these
parameters.

In addition, if you enter a value for another RF parameter, it is directly passed
to the randomForest() function for all the RF built during the procedure. For
example, if we add the option maxnodes= 2 to the arguments of the VSURF()
function, the whole procedure is performed with trees with 2 leaves.

```
> vsurfToysStump <- VSURF(toys$x, toys$y, mtry = 100, maxnodes = 2)
> summary(vsurfToysStump)

  VSURF computation time: 31.3 secs

  VSURF selected:
      14 variables at thresholding step (in 27.2 secs)
      8 variables at interpretation step (in 3 secs)
      2 variables at prediction step (in 1.1 secs)
> vsurfToysStump$varselect.interp

  [1]   3   2   1   5   6 159  37 111
> vsurfToysStump$varselect.pred

  [1] 3 5
```

There are also parameters specific to VSURF():

- The number of trees in the forests for each of the three steps of the method:
  nfor.thres (which is the most important, because if it is taken too small, the
  estimated standard deviation at the thresholding step will be of bad quality; 50 by
  default), nfor.interp, and nfor.pred (25 by default, which stabilize the
  OOB error estimates for the last two steps).
- nmin (=**n**umber of **min**imum) sets the multiplying factor of the estimated standard
  deviation of the VI of a noise variable, to calculate the threshold value of the first
  step: "threshold = min × standard deviation of VI for noise variables". By default,
  it is set to 1, and increasing it amounts to a more restrictive thresholding and has
  the consequence of keeping fewer variables after the first step.
- nsd (=**n**umber of **s**tandard **d**eviation) allows to apply the rule "nsd SE rule"
  instead of applying the rule "1-SE rule" (introduced in Sect. 2.3). We would select
  fewer variables for the "interpretation" if we increase this value.

- `nmj` (=**n**umber of **m**ean **j**ump) is the multiplying factor of the mean jump due to the inclusion of a noise variable in the nested models in the last step.

Two functions allow to adjust the thresholding and interpretation steps without having to perform all the calculations again.

- First of all, a `tune()` method which, applied to the result of `VSURF_thres()`, allows to set the thresholding step. The parameter `nmin` (whose default value is 1) can be used to set the threshold to the minimum prediction value given by the CART model multiplied by `nmin`.

```
> vsurfThresToysTuned <- tune(vsurfThresToys, nmin = 3)
> vsurfThresToysTuned$varselect.thres

 [1]   3   2   6   5   1   4 184  37 138  81 159  17 180 191
```

We get 16 selected variables instead of 36 previously.
- Second, a `tune()` method which, applied to the result of `VSURF_interp()`, is of the same type and allows to set the interpretation step. If we now want to be more restrictive in our selection in the interpretation step, we can select the smallest model with an OOB error lower than the minimum OOB error plus an empirical standard deviation multiplied by `nsd` (with $nsd \geq 1$).

```
> vsurfInterpToysTuned <- tune(vsurfInterpToys, nsd = 5)
> vsurfInterpToysTuned$varselect.interp

 [1] 3 2 6
```

We get 3 selected variables instead of 4 previously.

Finally, since the prediction step is a step-by-step process, to adjust this step, simply restart the `VSURF_pred()` function by changing the value of the parameter `nmj`.

```
> vsurfPredToysTuned <- VSURF_pred(toys$x, toys$y,
    err.interp = vsurfInterpToys$err.interp,
    varselect.interp = vsurfInterpToys$varselect.interp, nmj = 3)
> vsurfPredToysTuned$varselect.pred

 [1] 3 6 5
```

5.6 Examples

5.6.1 Predicting Ozone Concentration

For a presentation of this dataset, see Sect. 1.5.2.

```
> library(VSURF)
> data("Ozone", package = "mlbench")
```

After loading the data, the result of the entire selection procedure is obtained by using the following command:

```
> set.seed(303601)
> OzVSURF <- VSURF(V4 ~ ., data = Ozone, na.action = na.omit)
> summary(OzVSURF)

  VSURF computation time: 1.4 mins

  VSURF selected:
    9 variables at thresholding step (in 50.7 secs)
    5 variables at interpretation step (in 21.6 secs)
    5 variables at prediction step (in 9.8 secs)
```

```
> plot(OzVSURF, var.names = TRUE)
```

Let us now examine these results successively (illustrated in Fig. 5.4). To reflect the order used in the definition of the variables, we first reorganize the variables at the end of the procedure.

```
> number <- c(1:3, 5:13)
> number[OzVSURF$varselect.thres]
  [1]  9  8 12  1 11 10  5  7 13
```

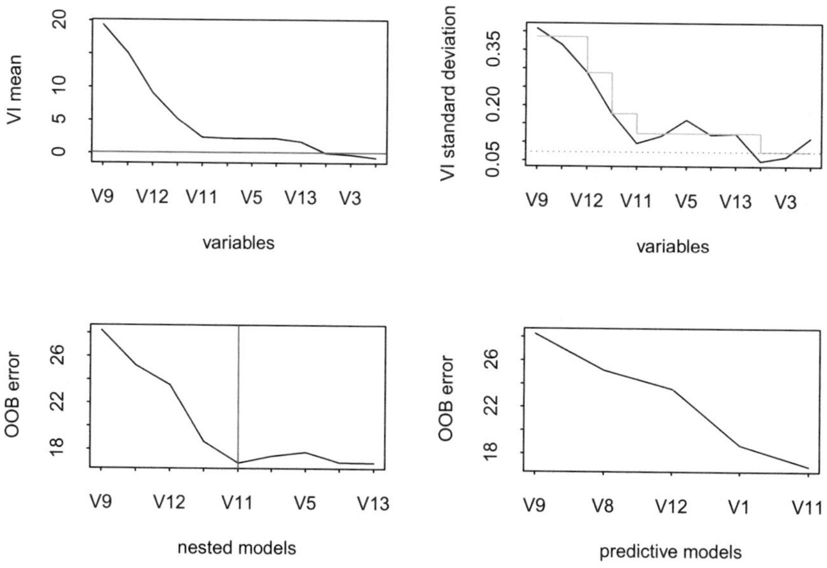

Fig. 5.4 Illustration of the results of VSURF(), Ozone data

After the first step, the 3 variables of negative importance (variables 6, 3, and 2) are eliminated as expected.

```
> number[OzVSURF$varselect.interp]
  [1]  9  8 12  1 11
```

Then, the interpretation procedure leads to the selection of the 5-variable model, which contains all the most important variables.

```
> number[OzVSURF$varselect.pred]
  [1]  9  8 12  1 11
```

With the default settings, the prediction step does not remove any additional variables.

In fact, our strategy more or less assumes that there exist some useless variables in the set of all initial variables, which is indeed the case in this dataset but not very significantly.

In addition, it should be noted here that our heuristics are clearly driven by prediction since the criterion for assessing the interest of a variable is closely related to the quality of the prediction or more exactly to its increasing after permutation.

5.6.2 Analyzing Genomic Data

For a presentation of this dataset, see Sect. 1.5.3.

Let us load the **VSURF** package, the `vac18` data, and then create an object `geneExpr` containing the gene expressions and an object `stimu` containing the stimuli to be predicted:

```
> library(VSURF)
> data("vac18", package = "mixOmics")
> geneExpr <- vac18$genes
> stimu <- vac18$stimulation
```

The global procedure with all parameters set to default values (note that the default value of `mtry` is $p/3$ even in classification, because as we have seen previously, the value of this parameter must be relatively high for high-dimensional problems) is obtained as follows:

```
> set.seed(481933)
> vacVSURF <- VSURF(x = geneExpr, y = stimu)
> summary(vacVSURF)
  VSURF computation time: 3.1 mins
```

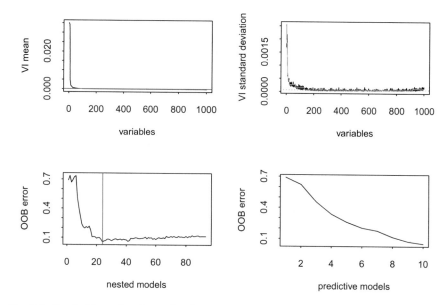

Fig. 5.5 Graphs illustrating the results of VSURF(), Vac18 data

```
VSURF selected:
    93 variables at thresholding step (in 1.7 mins)
    24 variables at interpretation step (in 1.3 mins)
    10 variables at prediction step (in 7.9 secs)
> plot(vacVSURF)
```

The first thresholding step keeps only 93 variables. This is reasonable given the graph of the importance of the variables located at the top left of Fig. 5.5, which as pointed out in Sect. 4.5.3, illustrates a strong parsimony in the Vac18 data.

The interpretation step of VSURF() leads to the selection of 24 variables, while the prediction step selects 10 variables.

Finally, the names of the variables (identifiers of the biochip probes used to measure gene expression) selected in the prediction step can be extracted as follows:

```
> probeSelPred <- colnames(geneExpr)[vacVSURF$varselect.pred]
> probeSelPred

  [1] "ILMN_1691156" "ILMN_2124802" "ILMN_2102693" "ILMN_1736939"
  [5] "ILMN_3252733" "ILMN_2188204" "ILMN_1658396" "ILMN_1663032"
  [9] "ILMN_3301824" "ILMN_2067444"
```

Computing time

The VSURF() function can be run in parallel using the following command:

```
> set.seed(627408, kind = "L'Ecuyer-CMRG")
> vacVSURFpara <- VSURF(x = geneExpr, y = stimu, parallel = TRUE,
    ncores = 3, clusterType = "FORK")
> summary(vacVSURFpara)
```

```
VSURF computation time: 1.5 mins

VSURF selected:
    97 variables at thresholding step (in 45.9 secs)
    23 variables at interpretation step (in 38 secs)
    13 variables at prediction step (in 7 secs)

VSURF ran in parallel on a PSOCK cluster and used 3 cores
```

We observe in this example a factor of about 2 in terms of saving execution time by using 3 cores instead of 1.

References

Alfaro, E., Gámez, M., & García, N. (2013). adabag: An R package for classification with boosting and bagging. *Journal of Statistical Software, 54*(2), 1–35.

Archer, K. J., & Kimes, R. V. (2008). Empirical characterization of random forest variable importance measures. *Computational Statistics and Data Analysis, 52*(4), 2249–2260.

Azen, R., & Budescu, D. V. (2003). The dominance analysis approach for comparing predictors in multiple regression. *Psychological Methods, 8*(2), 129.

Bach, F. R. (2008). Bolasso: model consistent lasso estimation through the bootstrap. In *Proceedings of the 25th international conference on machine learning* (pp. 33–40). ACM.

Biau, G. (2012). Analysis of a random forests model. *Journal of Machine Learning Research, 13*(38), 1063–1095.

Bobbia, M., Jollois, F.-X., Poggi, J.-M., & Portier, B. (2011). Quantifying local and background contributions to PM10 concentrations in Haute-Normandie, using random forests. *Environmetrics, 22*(6), 758–768.

Boulesteix, A.-L., Janitza, S., Kruppa, J., & König, I. R. (2012). Overview of random forest methodology and practical guidance with emphasis on computational biology and bioinformatics. *Wiley Interdisciplinary Reviews: Data Mining and Knowledge Discovery, 2*(6), 493–507.

Breiman, L. (1996). Bagging predictors. *Machine Learning, 24*(2), 123–140.

Breiman, L. (1998). Arcing classifier. *The Annals of Statistics, 26*(3), 801–849.

Breiman, L. (2000). Randomizing outputs to increase prediction accuracy. *Machine Learning, 40*(3), 229–242.

Breiman, L. (2001). Random forests. *Machine Learning, 45*(1), 5–32.

Breiman, L., & Friedman, J. H. (1985). Estimating optimal transformations for multiple regression and correlation. *Journal of the American Statistical Association, 80*(391), 580–598.

Breiman, L., Friedman, J., Olshen, R., & Stone, C. (1984). *Classification and regression trees*. New York: Chapman and Hall.

Cadenas, J. M., Carmen Garrido, M., & Martínez, R. (2013). Feature subset selection filter-wrapper based on low quality data. *Expert Systems with Applications, 40*(16), 6241–6252.

Chen, C., Liaw, A., & Breiman, L. (2004). *Using random forest to learn imbalanced data* (Vol. 110, pp. 1–12). Berkeley: University of California.

Core Team, R. (2018). *R: A Language and Environment for Statistical Computing*. Vienna, Austria: R Foundation for Statistical Computing.

Cutler, A. (2010). Remembering Leo Breiman. *The Annals of Applied Statistics, 4*(4), 1621–1633.

© Springer Nature Switzerland AG 2020
R. Genuer and J.-M. Poggi, *Random Forests with R*, Use R!,
https://doi.org/10.1007/978-3-030-56485-8

Díaz-Uriarte, R., & Alvarez De Andres, S. (2006). Gene selection and classification of microarray data using random forest. *BMC Bioinformatics*, *7*(1), 3.

Dietterich, T. G. (2000). Ensemble methods in machine learning. *International workshop on multiple classifier systems* (pp. 1–15). Berlin: Springer.

Fan, J., & Lv, J. (2008). Sure independence screening for ultrahigh dimensional feature space. *Journal of the Royal Statistical Society: Series B (Statistical Methodology)*, *70*(5), 849–911.

Fellinghauer, B., Bühlmann, P., Ryffel, M., Von Rhein, M., & Reinhardt, J. D. (2013). Stable graphical model estimation with random forests for discrete, continuous, and mixed variables. *Computational Statistics and Data Analysis*, *64*, 132–152.

Fernández-Delgado, M., Cernadas, E., Barro, S., & Amorim, D. (2014). Do we need hundreds of classifiers to solve real world classification problems. *Journal of Machine Learning Research*, *15*(1), 3133–3181.

Freund, Y., & Schapire, R. E. (1997). A decision-theoretic generalization of on-line learning and an application to boosting. *Journal of Computer and System Sciences*, *55*(1), 119–139.

Friedman, J. H. (1991). Multivariate adaptive regression splines. *The Annals of Statistics*, 1–67.

Genuer, R., Michel, V., Eger, E., & Thirion, B. (2010a). Random forests based feature selection for decoding fMRI data. In *Proceedings COMPSTAT* (Vol. 267, pp. 1–8).

Genuer, R., Poggi, J.-M., & Tuleau-Malot, C. (2018). VSURF: Variable Selection Using Random Forests. *R package version*, *1*, 4.

Genuer, R., Poggi, J.-M., & Tuleau, C. (2008). Random forests: some methodological insights. arXiv:0811.3619.

Genuer, R., Poggi, J.-M., & Tuleau-Malot, C. (2010b). Variable selection using random forests. *Pattern Recognition Letters*, *31*(14), 2225–2236.

Genuer, R., Poggi, J.-M., & Tuleau-Malot, C. (2015). VSURF: An R package for variable selection using random forests. *The R Journal*, *7*(2), 19–33.

Gey, S. (2002). *Bornes de risque, détection de ruptures, boosting: trois thèmes statistiques autour de CART en régression*. Ph.D. thesis, Paris 11, Orsay.

Ghattas, B. (1999). Prévisions des pics d'ozone par arbres de régression, simples et agrégés par bootstrap. *Revue de Statistique Appliquée*, *47*(2), 61–80.

Ghattas, B. (2000). Agrégation d'arbres de classification. *Revue de Statistique Appliquée*, *48*(2), 85–98.

Ghattas, B., & Ben Ishak, A. (2008). Sélection de variables pour la classification binaire en grande dimension: comparaisons et application aux données de biopuces. *Journal de la Société Française De Statistique*, *149*(3), 43–66.

Giraud, C. (2014). *Introduction to high-dimensional statistics*, (Vol. 138). CRC Press.

Goldstein, B. A., Hubbard, A. E., Cutler, A., & Barcellos, L. F. (2010). An application of random forests to a genome-wide association dataset: methodological considerations and new findings. *BMC Genetics*, *11*(1), 1.

Gregorutti, B. (2016). RFgroove: Importance Measure and Selection for Groups of Variables with Random Forests. *R package version*, *1*, 1.

Gregorutti, B., Michel, B., & Saint-Pierre, P. (2013). Correlation and variable importance in random forests. *Statistics and Computing*, 1–20.

Gregorutti, B., Michel, B., & Saint-Pierre, P. (2015). Grouped variable importance with random forests and application to multiple functional data analysis. *Computational Statistics and Data Analysis*, *90*, 15–35.

Grömping, U. (2015). Variable importance in regression models. *Wiley Interdisciplinary Reviews: Computational Statistics*, *7*(2), 137–152.

Guyon, I., Weston, J., Barnhill, S., & Vapnik, V. (2002). Gene selection for cancer classification using support vector machines. *Machine Learning*, *46*(1–3), 389–422.

Hapfelmeier, A., & Ulm, K. (2012). A new variable selection approach using random forests. *Computational Statistics and Data Analysis*, *60*, 50–69.

Ho, T. K. (1998). The random subspace method for constructing decision forests. *IEEE Transactions on Pattern Analysis and Machine Intelligence*, *20*(8), 832–844.

Hothorn, T., Hornik, K., Strobl, C., and Zeileis, A. (2017). *party: A Laboratory for Recursive Partytioning.* R package version 1.2–3.

Hothorn, T., Bühlmann, P., Dudoit, S., Molinaro, A., & Van Der Laan, M. J. (2006). Survival ensembles. *Biostatistics, 7*(3), 355–373.

Ishwaran, H., & Kogalur, U. (2017). Random Forests for Survival, Regression, and Classification (RF-SRC). *R package version, 2*(5), 1.

Ishwaran, H., Kogalur, U. B., Blackstone, E. H., & Lauer, M. S. (2008). Random survival forests. *The Annals of Applied Statistics,* 841–860.

Jollois, F.-X., Poggi, J.-M., & Portier, B. (2009). Three non-linear statistical methods for analyzing PM10 pollution in Rouen area. *Case Studies In Business, Industry and Government Statistics, 3*(1), 1–17.

Karatzoglou, A., Smola, A., Hornik, K., & Zeileis, A. (2004). kernlab–an S4 package for kernel methods in R. *Journal of Statistical Software, 11*(9), 1–20.

Kass, G. V. (1980). An exploratory technique for investigating large quantities of categorical data. *Applied statistics,* 119–127.

Le Cao, K.-A., Rohart, F., Gonzalez, I., & with key contributors Benoit Gautier, S. D., Bartolo, F., contributions from Pierre Monget, Coquery, J., Yao, F., & Liquet., B., (2017). mixOmics: Omics Data Integration Project. *R package version, 6*(3), 1.

Lê Cao, K.-A., Gonçalves, O., Besse, P., & Gadat, S. (2007). Selection of biologically relevant genes with a wrapper stochastic algorithm. *Statistical Applications in Genetics and Molecular Biology, 6*(1),

Leisch, F. & Dimitriadou, E. (2010). *mlbench: Machine Learning Benchmark Problems.* R package version 2.1–1.

Liaw, A. & Wiener, M. (2018). *randomForest: Breiman and Cutler's Random Forests for Classification and Regression.* R package version 4.6–14.

Liaw, A., & Wiener, M. (2002). Classification and regression by randomForest. *R News, 2*(3), 18–22.

Loh, W.-Y. (2014). Fifty years of classification and regression trees. *International Statistical Review, 82*(3), 329–348.

Louppe, G., Wehenkel, L., Sutera, A., & Geurts, P. (2013). Understanding variable importances in forests of randomized trees. *Advances in Neural Information Processing Systems,* 431–439.

Meinshausen, N., & Bühlmann, P. (2010). Stability selection. *Journal of the Royal Statistical Society: Series B (Statistical Methodology), 72*(4), 417–473.

Milborrow, S. (2018). *rpart.plot: Plot 'rpart' Models: An Enhanced Version of 'plot.rpart'.* R package version 2.2.0.

Olshen, R. (2001). A conversation with Leo Breiman. *Statistical Science,* 184–198.

Patil, D. V., & Bichkar, R. (2012). Issues in optimization of decision tree learning: A survey. *International Journal of Applied Information Systems, 3*(5),

Peters, A. & Hothorn, T. (2017). *ipred: Improved Predictors.* R package version 0.9–6.

Poggi, J.-M. & Tuleau, C. (2006). Classification supervisée en grande dimension. application à l'agrément de conduite automobile. *Revue de Statistique Appliquée, 54*(4), 41–60.

Prasad, A. M., Iverson, L. R., & Liaw, A. (2006). Newer classification and regression tree techniques: Bagging and random forests for ecological prediction. *Ecosystems, 9*(2), 181–199.

Questier, F., Put, R., Coomans, D., Walczak, B., & Vander Heyden, Y. (2005). The use of CART and multivariate regression trees for supervised and unsupervised feature selection. *Chemometrics and Intelligent Laboratory Systems, 76*(1), 45–54.

Quinlan, J. R. (1993). *C4. 5: Programming for machine learning.* Morgan Kauffmann.

Rakotomamonjy, A. (2003). Variable selection using SVM-based criteria. *Journal of Machine Learning Research, 3,* 1357–1370.

Ramosaj, B. & Pauly, M. (2019). Asymptotic unbiasedness of the permutation importance measure in random forest models. arXiv:1912.03306.

Ripley, B. (2018). *tree: Classification and Regression Trees.* R package version 1.0–39.

Segal, M., & Xiao, Y. (2011). Multivariate random forests. *Wiley Interdisciplinary Reviews: Data Mining and Knowledge Discovery, 1*(1), 80–87.

Seligman, M. (2017). *Rborist: Extensible, Parallelizable Implementation of the Random Forest Algorithm*. R package version 0.1–7.

Strobl, C., Boulesteix, A.-L., Zeileis, A., & Hothorn, T. (2007). Bias in random forest variable importance measures: Illustrations, sources and a solution. *BMC Bioinformatics, 8*(1), 25.

Strobl, C., Boulesteix, A.-L., Kneib, T., Augustin, T., & Zeileis, A. (2008). Conditional variable importance for random forests. *BMC Bioinformatics, 9*(1), 307.

Therneau, T. & Atkinson, B. (2018). *rpart: Recursive Partitioning and Regression Trees*. R package version 4.1–13.

Thiébaut, R., Liquet, B., Hocini, H., Hue, S., Richert, L., Raimbault, M., et al. (2012). A new method for integrated analysis applied to gene expression and cytokines secretion in response to LIPO-5 vaccine in HIV-negative volunteers. *Retrovirology, 9*(Suppl 2), P121.

Tibshirani, R. (1996). Regression shrinkage and selection via the lasso. *Journal of the Royal Statistical Society: Series B (Statistical Methodology)*, 267–288.

Vapnik, V. (2013). *The nature of statistical learning theory*. Springer Science and Business Media.

Verikas, A., Gelzinis, A., & Bacauskiene, M. (2011). Mining data with random forests: A survey and results of new tests. *Pattern Recognition, 44*(2), 330–349.

Wallard, H. (2015). *Analyse des leviers. Effets de colinéarité et hiérarchisation des impacts dans les études de marché et sociales*. Ph.D. thesis, CNAM, Paris.

Welling, S. H., Refsgaard, H. H., Brockhoff, P. B., & Clemmensen, L. H. (2016). Forest floor visualizations of random forests. arXiv:1605.09196.

Weston, J., Elisseeff, A., Schölkopf, B., & Tipping, M. (2003). Use of the zero norm with linear models and kernel methods. *The Journal of Machine Learning Research, 3*, 1439–1461.

Wright, M. N. (2017). ranger: A Fast Implementation of Random Forests. *R package version*, (8),

Wu, X., Kumar, V., Quinlan, J. R., Ghosh, J., Yang, Q., Motoda, H., et al. (2008). Top 10 algorithms in data mining. *Knowledge and information systems, 14*(1), 1–37.

Index

© Springer Nature Switzerland AG 2020
R. Genuer and J.-M. Poggi, *Random Forests with R*, Use R!,
https://doi.org/10.1007/978-3-030-56485-8

Printed in the United States
By Bookmasters